OFFICE ORTHOPEDICS FOR PRIMARY CARE

Diagnosis and Treatment

OFFICE ORTHOPEDICS FOR PRIMARY CARE

Diagnosis and Treatment

Bruce Carl Anderson, M.D.

Clinical Associate Professor of Medicine
Oregon Health Sciences University
Portland, Oregon
Director, Medical Orthopedic Department
Sunnyside Medical Center
Portland, Oregon

W.B. SAUNDERS COMPANY

A Division of Harcourt Brace & Company

Philadelphia London Toronto Montreal Sydney Tokyo

W.B. SAUNDERS COMPANY
A Division of
Harcourt Brace & Company

The Curtis Center
Independence Square West
Philadelphia, Pennsylvania 19106

1- 96

Library of Congress Cataloging-in-Publication Data

Anderson, Bruce Carl.

Office orthopedics for primary care: diagnosis and treatment /
Bruce Carl Anderson.

p.   cm.

Includes bibliographical references.

ISBN 0–7216–4576–3

1. Orthopedics.   2. Primary care (Medicine)
   I. Title.   [DNLM: 1. Bone Diseases—diagnosis.
   2. Fractures—therapy.   3. Family Practice—methods.
   WE 141 A545o 1995]

RD732.A53 1994   617.3—dc20

DNLM/DLC   94–25753

Office Orthopedics for Primary Care: Diagnosis and Treatment   ISBN 0–7216–4576–3

Printed in the United States of America.

Last digit is the print number: 9   8   7   6   5   4   3

To my loving parents, Eva and Earl Anderson.

Preface

This book represents the cumulative experience of 12 years of teaching the principles of orthopedic medicine to the departments of internal medicine and family practice at the Oregon Health Sciences University in Portland, Oregon. It evolved from a 20-page mimeographed teaching manual with rough illustrations and very abbreviated text to its current form over the last 4 years. It served as an introduction to the diagnosis and treatment of common, outpatient, nonsurgical orthopedic conditions. The book has attempted to bring together clinically useful information from several subspecialties, including internal medicine, orthopedics, neurology, physical medicine, and rehabilitation medicine.

This book is intended to provide clarity on the treatment of the common outpatient orthopedic problems that are so prevalent in the everyday practice of the primary care clinician. Family practitioners, internal medicine specialists, nurse practitioners, and osteopathic and chiropractic physicians will find it a practical guide.

The book is divided into four sections, including the diagnosis and treatment guidelines of the 44 most common outpatient orthopedic problems, ten fractures most frequently encountered by primary care clinicians, home physical therapy exercises commonly used in the rehabilitation of these conditions, and the most frequently used braces, casts, and splints. The appendix contains tables of the dosages and strengths of the injectable cortisone derivatives, the NSAIDs, and calcium supplements.

This book is intended to be comprehensive, providing the practitioner with accurate and easily accessible information on diagnosis and treatment. The "step-care" treatment protocols, the physical therapy exercise sheets, the illustrations of the various braces, casts, and supports, and the detailed descriptions of local injection techniques allow the clinician to "office manage" 90 to 95% of the outpatient medical orthopedic problems. Treatment guidelines provide details on specific restrictions, the length of time immobilization is both efficacious and practical, the appropriate timing and anatomic details of local injection, and the extremely important post-treatment rehabilitation exercises. Although local corticosteroid injection has been emphasized, this book was not intended to be simply an "injection manual." Injection of corticosteroids can be exceedingly helpful but must not take the place of simpler, less invasive treatments. Local injection of tendons, bursae, ligaments, or joints is indicated when local musculoskeletal inflammation persists despite rest and restriction, appropriate immobilization, and physical therapy.

Acknowledgments

This book represents the outgrowth of 13 years of postresidency education and clinical experience that would not have been possible without the support and encouragement from many sources. I wish to thank all the members of the Department of Internal Medicine at Sunnyside Medical Center, and especially Dr. Ian MacMillan and Dr. Edward Stark for their abiding support in the early years. I wish to thank all the medical residents of the graduating classes of 1993 and 1994 at the Oregon Health Sciences University for their constant encouragement and critical appraisal. I must also thank Professor David Gilbert for his stimulation to excellence, his inspiration to examine clinical problems ever more deeply, and for his support to return to clinical research. Last, I wish to thank my loving wife Gwen, and my three children, Jeremy, Jennifer, and Ryan, for their patience and understanding for the many hours I spent writing, drawing and editing this and my other writings.

Contents

The 44 Most Common Outpatient Orthopedic Conditions

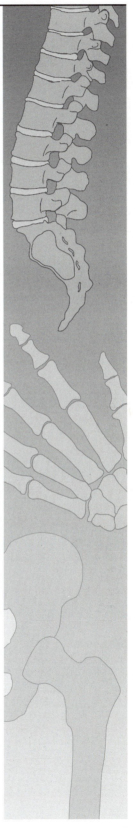

CHAPTER 1

Neck

CERVICAL STRAIN

Enter the upper trapezius muscle at the point of maximum tenderness; the angle is perpendicular to the skin.

Needle: 1 1/2", 22 gauge

Depth: 1 to 1 1/4"

Volume: 3 to 4 ml of 1% Xylocaine with or without 1 ml of D80

Note: lightly advance the needle to feel the outer fascia of the muscle; then enter the body of the muscle.

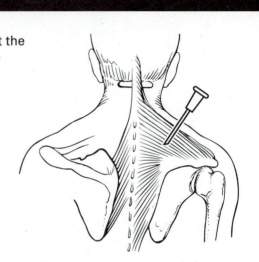

Figure 1–1. Cervical strain injection.

Description Cervical strain is an irritation and spasm of the upper back and cervical muscles. Physical and emotional stress, whiplash-like injuries, cervical arthritis, and underlying abnormal cervical alignment are common causes. The upper portion of the trapezius muscle and the levator scapulae, rhomboid major and minor, and the long cervical muscles are most often affected. Symptoms are bilateral in most cases. Several names are used to describe this condition, depending on etiology, chronicity, or anatomic predominance: neck strain, whiplash, trapezial strain, wry neck, torticollis, fibromyalgia, and fibrositis.

Symptoms Pain, stiffness, and tightness are described either in the upper back or shoulder.

"Oh, my aching neck."

"My neck is just a bunch of knots."

"My neck is so tight and tender."

"At the end of a hard day, my neck is so full of tension."

"My upper back feels like it has been tightened in a vise."

"If I sleep wrong, I wake up with a stiff neck and then I get this horrendous headache."

"My upper shoulder gets so stiff and tight."

Exam Each patient should be examined for the degree of spasm and specific points of irritation in the upper back and lower cervical muscles (referred to as "trigger points") and for the extent of loss of normal neck flexibility.

EXAM SUMMARY

1. Trigger points (upper back, paracervical, and rhomboids)
2. Reduced ipsilateral rotation and contralateral bending of the neck
3. Normal neurologic exam
4. No bony tenderness

(1) Trigger points are most frequently seen in the middle portion of the upper trapezius muscle, in the long cervical muscles at the base of the neck (at the C6–C7 vertebral level), and in the rhomboid muscles along the medial scapular border. The tenderness may be very localized to a small, quarter-sized area or may affect a diffuse area of muscle in chronic cases. (2) The range of motion of the neck may be limited, correlating well with the degree of muscle spasm. As muscle spasm increases, greater loss of ipsilateral neck rotation and of contralateral neck bending is seen. (Normal rotation of the neck is 90 degrees. Normal lateral bending is 45 degrees.) Flexion and extension of the neck are affected in extreme cases or in those with underlying arthritis. (3) The neurologic exam of the upper extremities is normal. (4) Bony structures of the neck, shoulder, and upper back are usually not tender.

X-Rays A cervical spine series with oblique views is recommended. Mild to moderate cases of cervical strain have normal x-ray appearance or nonspecific arthritic changes. Changes specific for cervical strain are seen only in moderate to severe cases! The normal cervical lordotic curve can be replaced by a straightened or even a reversed curve. These are best evaluated on the lateral view of the neck. Severe torticollis may cause a lateral deviation of the cervical spine, which is best seen on the posteroanterior view of the neck.

Diagnosis The diagnosis is based on a history and physical findings of localized upper back and neck tenderness, the characteristic aggravation of symptoms by ipsilateral rotation and contralateral bending of the neck, and the absence of evidence of radiculopathy by history or on exam. Plain films of the cervical spine are used to assess the severity of the condition and to exclude underlying bony pathology. Regional anesthetic block into a trigger point may be helpful in complex cases to help differentiate referred pain arising from an irritated cervical root or from subscapular bursitis at the superior medial angle of the scapula.

Treatment The goals of treatment are to reduce muscle irritability and spasm and to re-establish the normal cervical lordosis.

Step 1: Simple changes in lifestyle are suggested, including sitting straight with the shoulders held back, sleeping with the head and neck aligned with the body (a small pillow under the neck), driving with the arms slightly shrugged (arm rests), and avoiding straps over the shoulders. Heat and massage are applied to the upper back and to the base of the neck (p. 143).

Stress reduction is discussed. Gentle stretch exercises are performed daily, including shoulder rolls, scapular pinch, and neck stretches (p. 142). A muscle relaxer is prescribed for nighttime use. Nonsteroidal anti-inflammatory drugs (NSAIDs) (e.g., ibuprofen [Advil, Motrin]) are probably of little benefit (inflammation does not play a prominent role!).

Step 2 (3 to 4 weeks): An x-ray film of the neck is taken. An ultrasound treatment is done, and deep massage is given by a physical therapist. Gentle cervical traction is applied, beginning at 5 lb for 5 to 10 minutes once a day (p. 143). A soft cervical collar is used during physical work (p. 168).

Step 3 (6 to 8 weeks): A local trigger point injection is given with a local anesthetic, with or without a long-acting corticosteroid (for acute exacerbations). A tricyclic antidepressant is given for long-term control of pain. Referral is made to a transcutaneous electrical nerve stimulator (TENS) unit or to a pain clinic.

Physical Therapy Physical therapy is fundamental in the treatment and prevention of cervical strain.

PHYSICAL THERAPY SUMMARY

1. Muscular stretching exercises
2. Stretching plus heat and a muscle relaxer
3. Deep muscle massage
4. Ultrasound
5. "Gentle" vertical cervical traction

ACUTELY   Heat, massage, and gentle stretch exercises are used to reduce muscular irritation. These exercises should be performed daily at home. *Heat and massage* to the upper back and to the base of the neck provide temporary relief of pain and spasm. These can be combined with a nighttime muscle relaxer for greater effects. *Stretching exercises* are always recommended to regain flexibility and to counteract muscular spasm (p. 142). Heat and a muscle relaxer may enhance the effects of stretching. More advanced or protracted cases may need *deep pressure massage* or *ultrasound treatment* from a licensed therapist.

RECOVERY/REHABILITATION   Muscular stretching exercises and cervical traction are used to treat persistent or chronic cases. *Stretching exercises* must be continued three times a week to maintain neck flexibility. Chronic cases benefit from gentle *cervical traction,* beginning with a low weight of 5 to 10 lb for 5 minutes once or twice a day (p. 143). Note that severely irritated cervical muscles must be stretched cautiously. Traction can be irritating if applied too long, too frequently, or at too heavy a weight. Assess the patient's tolerance to traction by applying vertical traction in the office, either by manual traction or with a cervical traction unit.

Injection Technique   Local injection is adjunctive at best. It should be reserved for acute exacerbations.

Position: The patient sits up with the shoulders held back. The hands are placed in the lap.

Technique: The point of maximum tenderness is palpated. A local anesthetic or a corticosteroid is injected down to and into the belly of the muscle. The depth is rarely over 1 to 1¼". To determine the depth of injection, either use local anesthesia at ½" intervals or lightly advance the needle in order to feel the outer fascial covering of the muscle. Place 1 ml of anesthetic just outside the muscle; wait 1 to 2 minutes, and then penetrate the muscle. Distribute the volume in an area that is the size of a quarter with three punctures into the muscle.

Restrictions: Do not exceed three treatments per year! Repeated punctures into the same area can cause bleeding, fibrosis, atrophy, or contracture of the muscle! Avoid ultrasound and deep massage for several days. Begin gentle stretch exercises on day 4.

Prognosis   Cervical strain is a universal problem. Symptoms frequently recur. Fibromyalgia probably represents a more extensive process. Surgery is not applicable.

CERVICAL RADICULOPATHY

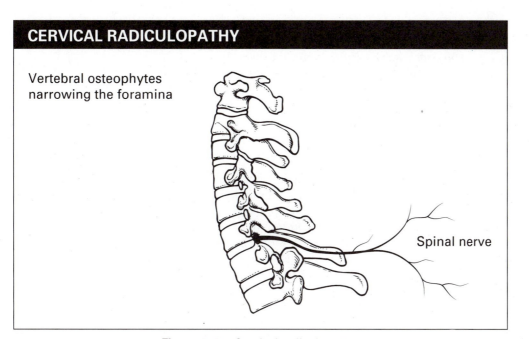

Vertebral osteophytes narrowing the foramina

Spinal nerve

Figure 1–2. Cervical radiculopathy.

Description Cervical radiculopathy is an impairment of the upper extremity neurologic function due to an abnormal process in the neck. Cervical arthritis with foraminal encroachment and a herniated nucleus pulposus are the two most common causes. Increasing irritation and pressure over the cervical root leads to progressive nerve impairment: sensory loss, loss of deep tendon reflexes, loss of motor strength, tone, or bulk, or in severe cases, long tract symptoms.

Symptoms Most patients have numbness or tingling in selected fingers. A few patients describe an electric-like pain over the scapula or radiating from the base of the neck down the arm. Advanced cases may be associated with loss of grip strength or lifting or pushing capacity.

"My fingers feel like they are coming out of Novocain."

"My hand feels numb."

"I think that I have a pinched nerve."

"I have shooting pains down my arm that feel like someone is driving nails into the muscles of my arm."

"It's like your foot goes to sleep—like the nerve is coming out of it."

"I was working on a ladder, and when I looked straight up, I felt this electric shock in the base of my neck."

"I've been dropping things."

Exam Each patient should be examined for the degree of muscle irritability in the upper back and neck, for the extent of loss of normal neck flexibility, and for abnormalities on the upper extremity neurologic exam.

EXAM SUMMARY

> 1. Abnormal upper extremity neurologic exam
> 2. Loss of full rotation of the neck and limited extension
> 3. A positive Spurling sign
> 4. Vertical traction may or may not afford relief
> 5. Paracervical tenderness

(1) Findings on the upper extremity neurologic exam are abnormal. Two-point discrimination, light touch, or pinprick sensation may be lost in selective fingers. Deep tendon reflexes may be asymmetric. Grip, biceps, or triceps strength may be impaired in advanced cases. Note that it is important to test strength two or three times to assess the power reserve of the muscle groups. (2) The neck often lacks full range of motion, especially in rotation and extension. (Normal rotation of the neck is 90 degrees.) The loss of rotation correlates directly with the degree of underlying arthritis or the degree of secondary muscular irritation. (3) Nerve root irritation can be brought out by 10 seconds of pressure or by tapping over the top of the cranium (Spurling maneuver) or (4) improved by neck traction applied by the examiner's hands. (5) Signs of cervical strain may be present (p. 4).

X-Rays   A cervical spine series is always recommended. Plain films of the neck may show a loss of the normal cervical lordosis or foraminal encroachment (nearly 90% of cervical radiculopathy is caused by hypertrophic spur nerve root compression at the foraminal level). Because spur formation can occur at multiple levels, the neurologic findings must be correlated with the radiographic abnormalities. For example, symptoms and signs involving the fifth root should correlate with the radiographic changes of foraminal encroachment at vertebral level C5–C6! A magnetic resonance imaging (MRI) scan should be obtained when neurologic findings persist despite reasonable treatment and especially when the plain cervical films are normal.

Diagnosis   The diagnosis of cervical radiculopathy is based on the combination of a history of radicular pain and paresthesia, neurologic impairment on exam, and abnormalities on plain films of the neck or on MRI scan.

Treatment   The goals of treatment are to reduce pressure over the nerve, improve neurologic function, and improve neck flexibility.

Step 1: Order a neck x-ray film or MRI scan, depending on the severity of the symptoms. Recommend seat belts and an air bag.

> Advise on the proper posture.
>
> Advise on proper nighttime sleeping posture: the patient should sleep with the head and neck aligned with the body (using a small pillow under the neck when lying on the back or several pillows while lying on the side).
>
> Underscore the importance of stress reduction.
>
> Apply massage and heat to the upper neck and back (p. 143).
>
> Offer a nighttime muscle relaxer (daytime use of a muscle relaxer may aggravate the condition!).
>
> Offer a soft cervical collar (p. 168) or a Philadelphia collar for severe muscle irritability (p. 168).
>
> NSAIDs (e.g., ibuprofen [Advil, Motrin]) probably do not help the primary process.

Step 2 (2 to 3 weeks): Re-evaluate neurologic function. Gentle rotation of the neck and lateral bending in sets of 20 should be performed after heat is applied (p. 142).

> Apply vertical cervical traction. A physical therapist can initiate this type of therapy; however, daily traction will have to be performed by the patient

at home. A water bag cervical traction unit should be prescribed. Traction is begun at 5 lb for 5 minutes. At intervals of 7 days, the weight and timing are gradually increased to a maximum of 12 to 15 lb for 10 minutes twice a day (p. 143). Prescribe a stronger muscle relaxant.

Step 3 (4 to 6 weeks): Re-evaluate neurologic function.
        Maximize vertical cervical traction.
        Set up a neurosurgical consultation if symptoms persist.

Physical Therapy   Physical therapy plays an integral part in the treatment of cervical radiculopathy and in the prevention of arthritis of the neck.

PHYSICAL THERAPY SUMMARY

> **1.** Cautious muscular stretching exercises
> **2.** Cautious stretching plus heat and massage
> **3.** Avoid ultrasound
> **4.** Gradually increasing amounts of vertical cervical traction

ACUTELY   Heat, massage, and gentle muscular stretching exercises are used to reduce secondary muscular irritation. (All the treatments used for cervical strain can be applied to cervical radiculopathy, but with caution!)

Heat and massage to the upper back and the base of the neck provide temporary relief of pain and muscle spasm. These can be combined with a nighttime muscle relaxer for additional effects.

Stretching exercises to reduce reactive muscular irritation and spasm must be used carefully (p. 142). The extremes of rotation and lateral bending may irritate the nerve roots (especially in foraminal encroachment disease). The tolerance of neck stretching must be assessed in the office prior to home use! *Ultrasound* should probably be avoided. It may aggravate nerve impingement.

RECOVERY/REHABILITATION   After the acute irritation has subsided, stretching exercises are combined with vertical cervical traction. *Stretch exercises* are performed daily to maintain neck flexibility and to counteract muscular spasm. The hallmark of therapy is *vertical cervical traction*. Almost all cases of foraminal encroachment show slow improvement in symptoms with traction (often over 4 to 6 weeks). Patients with herniated disks, however, may not tolerate traction at all. Depending on the vertical pull, radicular symptoms from a herniated disk may actually worsen with traction!

Injection Technique   Local injection is not routinely performed. If cervical strain is present, local injection of the trapezius muscle can be performed (p. 4). Facet joint injections should be performed by a neurosurgeon or by an interventional radiologist.

Prognosis   Most patients with cervical radiculopathy have underlying foraminal encroachment. In only 10% of cases, radicular symptoms arise from herniated disks (by contrast, 90% of radicular symptoms in the lumbosacral spine arise from herniated disks). Medical therapy is successful in more than 90% of patients with foraminal disease. Response to traction may be slow, however. It is not unusual to require 4 to 6 weeks to resolve sensory or early motor neurologic symptoms. Patients with reflex loss or dramatic motor weakness have a poorer prognosis and deserve an early work-up with MRI scanning and occasionally an electromyogram. Patients with herniated disks tend to be more resistant to medical treatment. Patients with a poor response to conservative therapy or with advanced neurologic symptoms should be evaluated by MRI scanning and should be referred to a neurosurgeon.

Shoulder

ROTATOR CUFF TENDINITIS

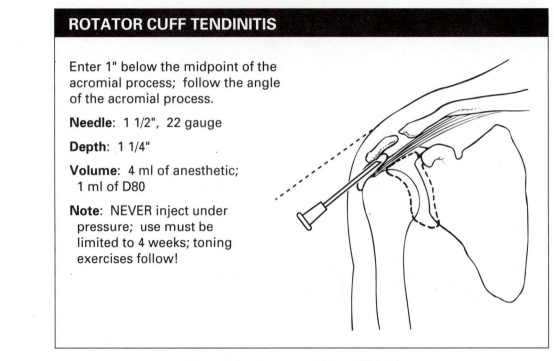

Enter 1" below the midpoint of the acromial process; follow the angle of the acromial process.

Needle: 1 1/2", 22 gauge

Depth: 1 1/4"

Volume: 4 ml of anesthetic; 1 ml of D80

Note: NEVER inject under pressure; use must be limited to 4 weeks; toning exercises follow!

Figure 2–1.   Subacromial bursal injection.

Description   Rotator cuff tendinitis is an inflammation of the supraspinatus and infraspinatus tendons lying between the humeral head and the acromial process. Overuse, when the arm is repeatedly abducted and elevated, leads to compression and irritation of the tendons (subacromial impingement). The subacromial bursa, located between the acromion and the two tendons, fails to provide sufficient lubrication and protection.

Symptoms   The patient has shoulder pain aggravated by overhead motions or restricted motion.

"Every time I reach over my head, I get this achy pain in my outer shoulder."

"I can't lift my arm over my head—it hurts so bad."

"I can't sleep on my shoulder! Every time I roll over in bed, my shoulder wakes me up."

"I can't reach up or back anymore."

"The only way I can stop the pain is to hang my arm over the side of the bed."

"Whenever I move suddenly or reach back, I get this sharp, deep pain in my shoulder."

Exam   Each patient should be examined for the degree of subacromial impingement and the degree of accompanying tendon inflammation.

EXAM SUMMARY

1. Focal subacromial tenderness
2. Subacromial "impingement," the painful arc maneuver
3. Pain with midarc abduction and external rotation
4. Normal range of motion of the glenohumeral joint
5. Preserved strength

(1) Subacromial tenderness is located between the greater tubercle of the humerus and the acromial process. Usually, this is very focal at the midacromion. (2) Impingement is assessed by the pain produced by passively abducting the arm (the painful arc). This maneuver compresses the swollen tendons and the subacromial bursa. (3) The degree of tendon inflammation is assessed by reproducing the patient's pain when resisting midarc abduction and external rotation isometrically. (4) Range of motion of the glenohumeral joint should be normal unless frozen shoulder has developed or underlying glenohumeral arthritis is present. (5) Abduction and external rotation strength should be normal in an uncomplicated case of tendinitis. If the patient's pain interferes with an accurate measurement of strength, a lidocaine injection test should be performed. The strength of the affected arm should be at least 75% of the strength of the unaffected side, unless a rotator cuff tendon tear is present.

X-Rays Routine x-rays of the shoulder are not always necessary. Calcification may be seen in approximately 30% of cases. A high-riding humeral head may indicate a large rotator cuff tendon tear (1%). Long-standing cases may have arthritic changes at the glenohumeral joint (<1%); however, with the exception of the latter two findings, the diagnosis and the decision to treat the patient rests on clinical grounds.

Cases accompanied by substantial weakness of midarc abduction or external rotation deserve either an arthrogram or magnetic resonance imaging (MRI) of the shoulder to evaluate for rotator cuff tear. Elderly patients older than 62 years of age who have suffered a fall to the outstretched arm or a direct blow to the shoulder are at increased risk or rotator cuff tendon rupture. Up to one third of 70 year olds with persistent symptoms have either a partial rotator cuff tendon rupture or a full-thickness rupture.

Diagnosis The diagnosis of rotator cuff tendinitis is based on the history of shoulder pain coupled with two of the three main signs on physical exam. The diagnosis is confirmed by regional anesthetic block in the subacromial bursa. Rotator cuff tendon ruptures can accompany rotator cuff tendinitis in 3 to 5% of cases. It is important to perform a lidocaine injection test to exclude an underlying rotator cuff tendon rupture prior to giving a local corticosteroid injection.

Treatment The goals of treatment are to reduce tendon swelling and inflammation, to increase the subacromial space thus reducing the degree of impingement, and to prevent progressive damage to the tendons.

Step 1: Rest and restriction of overhead positioning and reaching are suggested. Ice is given for acute pain. Weighted pendulum stretch exercises are performed using 5 to 10 lb for 5 minutes once or twice a day (p. 145).

Step 2 (2 to 4 weeks): A nonsteroidal anti-inflammatory drug (NSAID) (e.g., ibuprofen [Advil, Motrin]) is given in full dose for 3 to 4 weeks. Pendulum exercises are re-emphasized.

Simple arm slings are discouraged (p. 169). Immobilization in a susceptible patient (often with a low pain threshold) may hasten the development of frozen shoulder!

Step 3 (6 to 8 weeks): A lidocaine injection test is done to exclude a tendon tear. An arthrogram is done if the test result is abnormal (<50% pain relief and <75% of normal strength in abduction or external rotation); an MRI is taken if the patient has profound weakness and is a surgical candidate; or an ultrasound of the shoulder is taken if a trained technologist is available. A local injection of D80 is given if the patient has a normal lidocaine injection test result (>50% pain relief and >75% of normal strength).

Repeat the injection in 4 to 6 weeks if symptoms and signs have not decreased by at least 50%.

Step 4 (3 months): Weighted pendulum exercises plus toning exercises in abduction and external rotation are done to prevent a recurrence (pp. 145 to 146).

Reaching overhead is done cautiously.

Recurrent or persistent cases should avoid any repetitious overhead work or positioning!

An orthopedic consultation should be scheduled if symptoms persist or if the tendon has torn.

Physical Therapy   Physical therapy plays an active role in the early steps of treatment of rotator cuff tendinitis and serves an important role in the prevention of recurrent tendinitis.

PHYSICAL THERAPY SUMMARY

1. Ice
2. Weighted pendulum swing exercises
3. Toning exercises for the infraspinatus and supraspinatus tendons
4. Avoid simple slings or other shoulder immobilizers

ACUTELY   Ice and the weighted pendulum stretch exercises are used to reduce swelling and impingement. *Ice* in the form of a bag of frozen corn or an ice bag is used for temporary relief of pain and swelling. The *weighted pendulum swing exercise* is fundamental to stretching the subacromial space, allowing the rotator cuff tendons room to contract, and to aid in preventing frozen shoulder (p. 145). Initially, the subacromial space is stretched with the weight of the arm. With improvement a 5- to 10-lb weight is used as tolerated. It is exceedingly important to keep the arm vertical and relaxed when performing this exercise. Excessive bending at the waist may aggravate subacromial impingement. Active use of the shoulder muscles (as opposed to relaxing them) may aggravate the underlying tendon inflammation!

RECOVERY/REHABILITATION   The weighted pendulum swing exercises are continued through the recovery period, and the isometric toning exercises are begun 4 to 6 weeks after the acute pain and swelling has resolved. The *weighted pendulum swing exercise* is effective in preventing recurrent tendinitis. Maintenance exercises three times a week reduce the chance of recurrent tendon compression.

Isometric toning exercises of the infraspinatus and supraspinatus muscles are used to strengthen the weakened tendons, to stabilize the glenohumeral joint, and to open the subacromial space (p. 146). Preferential toning of the infraspinatus muscle has the theoretical advantage of increasing the distance between the humeral head and the acromion. These should be used 4 to 6 weeks after the acute symptoms have resolved in order to avoid inciting tendon inflammation.

Injection Technique   Local injection for uncomplicated rotator cuff tendinitis is indicated when restricted use, the pendulum stretch exercises, and a 3- to 4-week course of an NSAID fail to resolve the problem. One or two injections 6 weeks apart are safe and provide long-term control of symptoms in up to 90% of patients who consistently pass the lidocaine injection test.

Position: The patient is sat up, and the hands are placed in the lap. The patient is asked to relax the shoulder and neck muscles.

Technique: The lateral subacromial injection is safest. The tip of the acromion is identified. The needle is entered 1″ below the midpoint of the acromion and is angled up into the subacromial bursa, paralleling the acromial process. In a well-developed muscular patient a ''pop'' or giving way sensation is felt when the needle passes through the deep fascial covering of the deltoid. The needle is advanced to the hub, well under the acromial process. The lidocaine injection test is performed. Lidocaine is injected, and the shoulder is re-examined. If pain is significantly improved (50% or greater), and there is at least 75%

of normal strength in abduction and external rotation, then 1 ml of D80 is injected. All medication should be injected with light pressure (any resistance to an injection suggests a periosteal or intratendinous injection).

Restrictions: Minimal use of the shoulder and arm are recommended for 3 days. Ice is used for inflammatory flare reactions. Overhead reaching, pushing, pulling, and lifting are restricted for the next 30 days. Following recovery, isometric toning of abduction and external rotation are performed daily (p. 146).

Prognosis Of cases treated with one or two injections, 85 to 90% (6 weeks apart) do extremely well. Approximately one in three will recur, requiring retreatment in the next several years. Short- and long-term improvement, however, depend more on the degree of subacromial impingement, how well overhead work is avoided, and the degree of chronic degenerative change in the tendon. Surgery is indicated for chronic or persistent cases, with or without calcification or rotator cuff tendon tear. Primary tendon repair and excision of the calcific deposit can be combined with a procedure to reduce impingement (subacromial decompression or acromioplasty—the Neer procedure). Unfortunately, surgical treatment is only partially successful. Either procedure often improves the patient's pain but may not return the patient to the original level of function. Patients need to be advised that the success of surgery often depends on the degree of irreparable tendon damage and degeneration.

FROZEN SHOULDER

A frozen shoulder can be injected at the subacromial bursa (see rotator cuff tendinitis) or intra-articularly.

The intra-articular injection enters just below the coracoid and is directed outwardly.

Needle: 1 1/2", 22 gauge

Depth: 1"

Volume: 4 ml of anesthetic; 1 ml of D8O

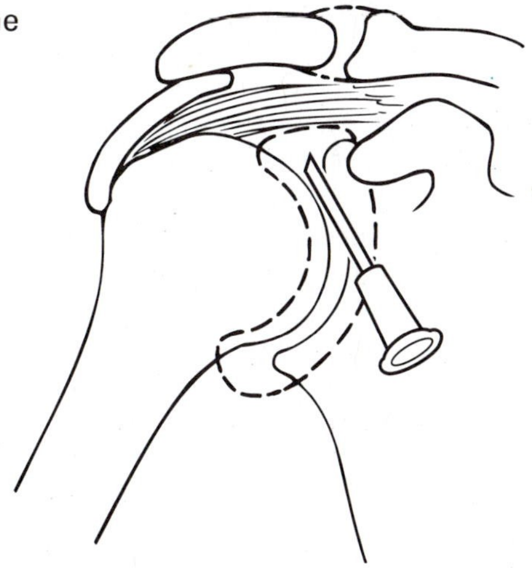

Figure 2–2. Frozen shoulder injection.

Description Frozen shoulder is a descriptive term referring to a stiff shoulder joint—a glenohumeral joint that has lost significant range of motion. Pathologically, the glenohumeral joint capsule has lost its normal distensibility. Long-standing cases may form adhesions between the joint capsule and the humeral head (adhesive capsulitis). Rotator cuff tendinitis, acute subacromial bursitis, fractures about the humeral head and neck, and paralytic stroke are common causes. Protracted cases with severe restriction of motion may be complicated by hand swelling, finger discoloration, Sudeck atrophy of bone, and pain up and down the arm (referred to as reflex sympathetic dystrophy or RSD).

Symptoms   The patient has a gradual loss of shoulder motion.

"I can't reach up over my head."

"I can't reach back to fasten my bra. I have to fasten it in front and rotate it around."

"My shoulder is stiffening up."

"I can't shave under my armpit anymore."

"My shoulder used to be quite sore and tender. The pain has gotten a lot better, but I can't move it now."

"It's getting harder and harder to put on my coat."

Exam   Each patient should be examined for loss of range of motion of the glenohumeral joint (especially in the directions of abduction and external rotation) along with the degree of inflammation arising from the periarticular structures.

EXAM SUMMARY

> 1. An abnormal Apley scratch test (inability to scratch the lower back)
> 2. Reduced abduction and external rotation (passively performed)
> 3. No x-ray evidence of glenohumeral arthritis
> 4. Hand swelling, finger discoloration, synovitis (RSD)

A general assessment of glenohumeral motion should be performed initially. This can be assessed by asking the patient to raise his or her arms overhead or by (1) the Apley scratch test. The latter can be used as a quick screening test for glenohumeral motion. Patients with normal glenohumeral motion should be able to scratch the midback at the T8-T10 vertebral level. Patients with frozen shoulder are unable to scratch even the lower back. (2) Next, individual motions should be measured. Passively measured abduction and external rotation are reduced most often. The glenohumeral joint should externally rotate to 90 degrees and abduct to 90 to 120 degrees. Note that in order to accurately measure abduction, shrugging must be prevented by placing downward pressure over the acromion. (3) Severe frozen shoulder, which lasts for many months, may be associated with diffuse hand pain and swelling, finger discoloration, abnormal patterns of sweating, or unilateral joint synovitis (reflex sympathetic dystrophy). (4) Advanced glenohumeral arthritis should be excluded by exam (arthritis will show loss of all ranges of motion) or by x-ray.

X-Rays   Special studies are not necessary to make this clinical diagnosis; however, routine plain films of the shoulder or even shoulder arthrography are obtained to exclude underlying glenohumeral arthritis (very infrequent) and to satisfy the patient's expectations (e.g., protracted symptoms, the patient's concern for an underlying process). Most plain films are nondiagnostic, although rotator cuff tendon calcification is found incidentally in 30% of cases. Shoulder arthrography may show characteristic changes of a contracted glenohumeral capsule. Normally, the glenohumeral joint fills with 7 or 8 ml of contrast. An advanced case of frozen shoulder may only accept 4 to 5 ml of contrast.

Diagnosis   The diagnosis is based on a persistent and reproducible loss of glenohumeral joint range of motion. Underlying glenohumeral arthritis needs to be excluded, preferably by routine x-ray. Occasionally, regional anesthetic block is necessary. A concomitant periarticular process may interfere with accurate glenohumeral motion measurements. The patient's periarticular pain may prevent full motion at the joint. Accurate measurements may not be possible until the patient's periarticular pain is reduced.

Treatment The goals of treatment are to treat any underlying periarticular or bony process, gradually stretch out the glenohumeral joint lining, and restore normal range of motion to the shoulder.

Step 1: Educate the patient about the slow recovery times. "This may take 6 to 18 months to recover."

Heat the anterior shoulder prior to stretching.

Pendulum stretch exercises daily (p. 145).

Passively performed stretch exercises in abduction and external rotation (p. 146).

Eliminate over-the-shoulder work in patients with signs of tendinitis.

An NSAID (e.g., ibuprofen [Advil, Motrin]) probably adds very little to treatment.

Step 2 (6 to 8 weeks): Re-evaluate the range of motion.

Reinforce the stretch exercises.

Consider a subacromial or intra-articular injection of D80.

Step 3 (3 months): Re-evaluate the range of motion.

Encourage the patient.

Step 4 (6 to 12 months): Gradually resume normal activities as motion improves.

Suggest pendulum stretch exercises to prevent a recurrence.

Consider intra-articular dilatation with lidocaine and saline.

Consider arthroscopic dilatation of the joint.

Use manipulation under anesthesia if symptoms fail to improve.

Physical Therapy Physical therapy is the principal treatment for frozen shoulder.

PHYSICAL THERAPY SUMMARY

1. Heat
2. Weighted pendulum exercises
3. Repetitive passive stretch exercises
4. Rotator cuff muscle toning (with underlying tendinitis)

ACUTELY/RECOVERY Heat, the weighted pendulum stretch exercises, and passive stretch exercises are used to restore glenohumeral flexibility. *Heat* is applied to the shoulder for 10 to 15 minutes either in a bathtub or shower or with moist heat.

Weighted pendulum stretch exercises are performed for 5 minutes (p. 145). The arm is kept vertical, slightly bending at the waist. Emphasis is placed on relaxing the shoulder muscles when instructing the patient. ("This is a pure stretch exercise." "Don't swing the weight greater than 1 foot in diameter." "Let the weight do the work.") *Passive stretch exercises* are performed after the pendulum stretch exercises. Emphasize stretch exercises in the direction that the patient has suffered the greatest loss, usually abduction and external rotation (p. 148). Limit the abduction stretch to no greater than shoulder level, if the frozen shoulder resulted from rotator cuff tendinitis. Emphasize the need to stretch to the point of tension and not pain. Multiple sets performed twice a day will gradually stretch the glenohumeral capsule. General *rotator cuff tendon toning* may play a minor role in recovery, especially if rotator cuff tendinitis preceded the frozen shoulder (p. 146).

Injection Technique A subacromial injection is indicated if there are signs of underlying rotator cuff tendinitis (p. 12). An intra-articular injection of D80 is indicated when simple passive stretch exercises fail to resolve the restricted range of motion. It may be prudent to perform an intra-articular injection under fluoroscopic control. Consultation with an orthopedist or a radiologist may be advisable.

Prognosis Frozen shoulder slowly improves over months. Loss of 50% or more of external rotation or abduction may be associated with permanent stiffness, especially in the diabetic patient; however, most patients recover fully. Surgical treatment is indicated for persistent or progressive loss of range of motion, despite reasonable conservative care. Arthroscopic dilatation has replaced the archaic manipulation under general anesthesia. These surgical procedures are indicated for the persistent case. Either procedure is used to break up adhesions that have formed over the humeral head.

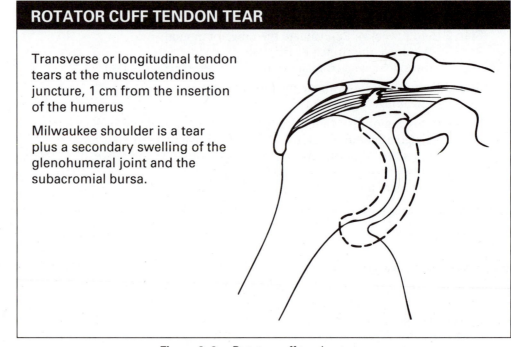

ROTATOR CUFF TENDON TEAR

Transverse or longitudinal tendon tears at the musculotendinous juncture, 1 cm from the insertion of the humerus

Milwaukee shoulder is a tear plus a secondary swelling of the glenohumeral joint and the subacromial bursa.

Figure 2–3.   Rotator cuff tendon tear.

Description A rotator cuff tendon tear is a loss of the normal integrity of the infraspinatus or supraspinatus tendons over the humeral head. Most occur in patients with underlying rotator cuff tendinitis. Tears can result from a fall to an outstretched arm or directly onto the outer shoulder, vigorous pulling on a lawn mower cable, or from the gradual attrition of chronic rotator cuff tendinitis. Tears are classified anatomically as tendon splits or transverse ruptures and functionally as "partial" or "complete."

Symptoms The patient has shoulder pain, weakness of the shoulder, or loss of smooth motion.

"I can't lift my arm up unless I push it up with my other arm."

"My shoulder has been sore for a long time. Yesterday, when I was lifting this heavy box, I felt a pop in my shoulder."

"I slipped on the ice and caught my fall with my arms. Ever since then my arm has been weak."

"I tried to start my lawn mower the other day. I pulled on the rope many times. The last time I pulled as hard as I could, and I felt this really sharp stabbing pain in my shoulder."

"That shot for my bursitis really took the pain away. I could finally get back to my gardening; however, when I was rototilling, my arm was jerked forward. It felt like a .22 shell went off in my shoulder. Now the pain is worse than ever."

Exam   Each patient should be examined for weakness of glenohumeral external rotation or abduction as well as for signs of active rotator cuff tendon inflammation.

EXAM SUMMARY

1. *Weakness* and pain of midarc abduction or external rotation
2. A painful arc of abduction (p. 13)
3. Subacromial tenderness
4. Loss of smooth overhead reaching
5. Atrophy of the infraspinatus or supraspinatus fossae

(1) The principal sign of a rotator cuff tendon tear is weakness of external rotation (infraspinatus) or midarc abduction (supraspinatus). Because this is most often a complication of rotator cuff tendinitis, weakness is accompanied by pain when testing the two tendons isometrically, (2) signs of subacromial impingement (the painful arc maneuver, see p. 13), and (3) local subacromial tenderness. Partial tears are distinguished by (4) a loss of smooth overhead reaching. Complete tears are distinguished by an inability to reach overhead, by anterior and superior migration of the humeral head, or rarely the drop arm sign. The drop arm sign is an inability to hold the upper extremity in midarc abduction. Long-standing cases (over several months) may show (5) atrophy of the infraspinatus or supraspinatus fossae over the scapula. Advanced cases with large tears may be associated with swelling of the subacromial bursa and the glenohumeral joint (referred to as Milwaukee shoulder).

X-Rays   Specialized testing is necessary to confirm the diagnosis. Arthrography will demonstrate most of the clinically significant tears. Dynamic ultrasound is a very accurate test but requires a trained technician. MRI scanning will demonstrate large transverse tears, those that are usually fairly obvious by clinical testing. MRI scanning may not differentiate the less obvious partial tear from ongoing tendinitis.

Diagnosis   The diagnosis of a rotator cuff tendon tear can be difficult. A high index of suspicion for tendon disruption should be kept in mind whenever rotator cuff tendinitis fails to improve with the standard stepped care or when there is a history of a fall to an outstretched arm or a history of heavy work (see earlier). Ultimately, if the clinical history, physical examination, or lidocaine injection test suggests a tear, then arthrography or MRI scanning should be performed.

Treatment   The goals of treatment are to resolve any concurrent tendinitis, to increase the subacromial space, to allow the split or torn tendon to heal, or to evaluate for possible surgery.

Step 1: Perform a subacromial bursa lidocaine injection test.

If the patient has persistent weakness in abduction or external rotation, or if minimal pain relief has been experienced, order an arthrogram or MRI scan.

Begin weighted pendulum swing exercises with 2 to 5 lb (less than that for rotator cuff tendinitis).

Perform daily toning exercises (p. 146).

Restrict over-the-shoulder work, pushing, pulling, and lifting over 10 lb.

An abduction pillow shoulder immobilizer, if tolerated, or a simple sling (p. 169) is combined with pendulum stretch exercises done three times a day.

Step 2 (4 to 6 weeks): Re-evaluate the patient's strength.
Continue toning and stretch exercises if the patient is improving.
Consider an orthopedic referral if the patient fails to improve.

Step 3 (8 to 10 weeks): Re-evaluate the patient's strength. Consider a subacromial injection of D80 for palliative pain relief in a nonsurgical candidate.

Physical Therapy   Physical therapy plays an important role in the active treatment of partial rotator cuff tendon tears and a significant role in the postoperative recovery of surgically repaired complete tears.

PHYSICAL THERAPY SUMMARY

> **1.** Heat
> **2.** Pendulum stretch exercises
> **3.** Isometric toning exercises of the rotator cuff muscles

ACUTELY/RECOVERY   Exercises to stretch the glenohumeral space are combined with toning exercises and restricted use. Daily *isometric toning exercises* of glenohumeral abduction and external rotation are essential to the rehabilitation of partial rotator cuff tendon tears (p. 146). These exercises are performed with low tension and high repetition using a TheraBand, large rubber bands, a spring tension chest expander, and so forth. Enough tension is used to stress the rotator cuff tendon muscles but not enough to aggravate an underlying tendinitis! The toning is enhanced if preceded by heating the shoulder for 10 to 15 minutes and by stretching the subacromial space with *weighted pendulum stretch exercises* (p. 145). These exercises are also very important to the overall success of the surgical repair of complete rotator cuff tendon tears.

Rehabilitation   General care of the shoulder coupled with a long-term restriction of overhead work is necessary to prevent further tendon deterioration. Emphasis is placed on the *weighted pendulum stretch exercises* and on *isometric toning exercises.*

Injection Technique   Moderate-to-large rotator cuff tendon tears with persistent pain and functional loss should be treated surgically. A local corticosteroid injection is recommended only for the nonsurgical candidate who has not responded to conservative physical therapy. Note that corticosteroid injection may worsen the underlying tendon.

Position: The patient is sat up, and the shoulders are held back. The hands are placed in the lap.

Technique: See Rotator Cuff Tendinitis (p. 14).

Restrictions: Minimal use of the shoulder and arm is recommended for 3 days. An abduction pillow immobilizer should be used for patients with significant weakness greater than 50%. Ice is used for inflammatory flares. Overhead reaching, pushing and pulling, and lifting are avoided for the next 30 days. At 4 weeks, isometric toning exercises are combined with daily pendulum swing exercises with weights (pp. 145 to 146).

Prognosis   A split or rupture of the rotator cuff tendon can result from a fall, lifting excessive amounts of weight, violent pulls on a starter cable, or excessive pushing and pulling. Minor tears with loss of only 25 to 50% of strength can be treated medically with exercises over many months. At least 50% of all tears heal with stretch exercises, toning, proper protection, and in selected cases a subacromial bursal injection of D80. Patients who do not respond to 4 weeks of conservative care should be promptly referred to the orthopedic surgeon. Unnecessary delays in surgery may lead to muscle atrophy, making recovery more difficult and prolonged. All patients should be warned that sharp dissection of large tears often leads to postoperative stiffness or to loss of range of motion.

ACROMIOCLAVICULAR STRAIN-OSTEOARTHRITIS

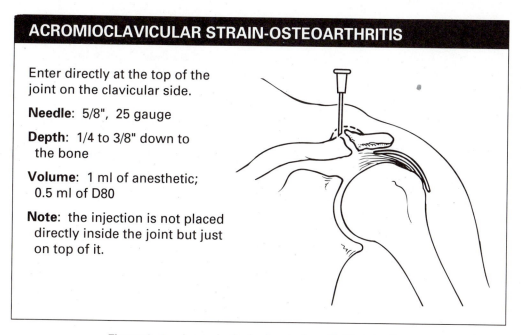

Enter directly at the top of the joint on the clavicular side.

Needle: 5/8", 25 gauge

Depth: 1/4 to 3/8" down to the bone

Volume: 1 ml of anesthetic; 0.5 ml of D80

Note: the injection is not placed directly inside the joint but just on top of it.

Figure 2–4. Acromioclavicular strain-arthritis injection.

Description   The acromioclavicular (AC) joint and its supporting ligaments are susceptible to injury by overuse and trauma. The AC, the coracoclavicular, and the coracoacromial ligaments, binding the acromion, clavicle and coracoid process together, can be strained, partially torn, or completely disrupted. This leads to a 1-degree, a 2-degree, or a 3-degree separation, respectively. Repeated strain or injury to the supporting ligaments may progress to osteoarthritis of the AC joint.

Symptoms   The patient complains of shoulder pain or swelling at the AC joint. The symptoms are often so localized that the patient points to the end of the collar bone with the index finger.

''Whenever I reach up or across my shoulder, I get a pain right here (pointing to the AC joint).''

''I fell off my mountain bike and landed right on my shoulder. Ever since then I have had achy pain and swelling right here (pointing to the AC joint).''

''If I reach up, I feel a grinding in my shoulder.''

''The bones seem to be rubbing against one another.''

''I can't lie on my shoulder. Sharp pain will wake me up.''

Exam   Each patient should be examined for joint inflammation, arthritic change, or disruption of the ligaments that support the joint.

EXAM SUMMARY

1. AC joint enlargement or deformity
2. AC joint tenderness (with or without swelling)
3. Pain aggravated by downward traction or forced passive adduction
4. AC joint widening with traction

(1) By simple inspection the AC joint may be distorted by tissue swelling, bony osteophytes, or elevation of the clavicle (3-degree separation). (2) Local tenderness (the most common symptom) is located at the top of the joint, approximately 1½″ from the lateral tip of the acromion. (3) Pain is most consistently aggravated by passively adducting the arm across the chest and by forcing the end of the clavicle and the acromial process together. (4) Also, pain may be aggravated by placing downward traction on the arm. In 2-degree and 3-degree separations, this may be accompanied by a widening of the gap between the clavicle and the acromion (palpable or visible in asthenic individuals or high-grade separations). (5) The diagnosis is supported by a local anesthetic block placed just over the joint.

X-Rays   Plain films and weighted views of the shoulder are recommended. Plain films of the shoulder may show degenerative change (e.g., narrowing, sclerosis, squaring off of the clavicle or acromion, or spurring). Weighted views of the shoulder (with and without hand-held weights) may show excessive widening between the end of the clavicle and the acromial process (>5 mm).

Treatment   The goal of treatment is to allow the ligament(s) to reattach to their respective bony insertions.

Step 1: Avoid sleeping on either side.
Do not reach overhead or across the chest.
Limit lifting to 10 to 20 lb, held close to the body.
Apply ice.
Use a shoulder immobilizer for 3 to 4 weeks (p. 170).
Educate the patient, "If the ligament isn't allowed to reattach to the bone, symptoms may recur over and over."

Step 2 (2 to 4 weeks): X-ray both shoulders (with and without weights) to distinguish first-, second-, and third-degree strains.
Re-emphasize the restriction.
Consider a local injection with D80, especially if swelling is prominent.
A second injection can be combined with a Velcro shoulder immobilizer for optimal protection (p. 170).

Step 3 (8 to 10 weeks): Consider an orthopedic referral for palliative surgery.

Physical Therapy   Physical therapy plays a minor role in the treatment of AC strain and degenerative arthritis of the AC joint. Ice over the AC joint can provide temporary symptomatic relief. Unfortunately, there are no effective isometric toning exercises or stretch exercises that will provide additional support to the joint.

Injection Technique   Immobilization and protection are the preferred treatments for this mechanical condition. Local injection is palliative at best, providing temporary relief.

Position: The patient is sat up, with the shoulders held back. The hands are placed in the lap.

Technique: Since the AC joint is too small to inject into directly, the medication is injected either on top of the joint or just under the synovial lining on the adjacent bone. The distal end of the clavicle is identified, and the needle is advanced vertically down to the bone. After identifying the depth of the bone, the needle is withdrawn 3 to 4 mm, and the local anesthetic is injected just outside the joint. Then, advance the needle back to the firm resistance of the bone. With the needle held flush against the bone, the corticosteroid is injected just under the synovial lining with gentle pressure. Inject the medication slowly but firmly. The joint will not accommodate much medication. If the patient has too much discomfort, stop the injection. Use only enough local anesthetic to confirm the diagnosis and provide local relief.

Restrictions: Overhead reaching, reaching across the chest, and sleeping directly on the shoulder are avoided for 3 days and are limited for the ensuing 30 days. For maximum benefit, a shoulder immobilizer can be used to prevent any aggravation caused by shoulder motion.

Prognosis Success of medical treatment is determined by adequate and anatomic healing of the injured ligaments. The emphasis of treatment must be on immobilization rather than on the anti-inflammatory action of injection. Unfortunately, since proper reattachment of the ligaments does not always occur, recurrent injury is seen frequently. Surgical consultation can be considered in recurrent cases, although immobilization with internal fixation is performed infrequently.

BICEPS TENDINITIS

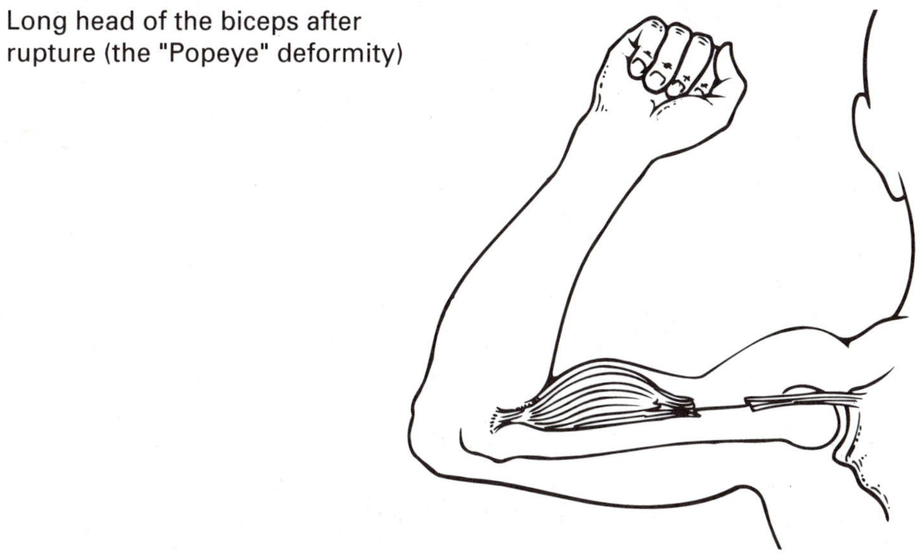

Long head of the biceps after rupture (the "Popeye" deformity)

Figure 2–5. Biceps tendinitis and rupture.

Description Biceps tendinitis is an inflammation of the long head tendon as it passes through the bicipital groove of the anterior humerus. Repeated irritation leads to microtearing and degenerative change. Vigorous lifting in a chronically inflamed tendon can lead to spontaneous rupture. The risk of rupture approaches 10 to 12%, which is the highest spontaneous rupture rate of any tendon in the body.

Symptoms The patient has shoulder pain (pointing to the front of the shoulder) aggravated by lifting or overhead pushing and pulling.

"The front of my shoulder hurts every time I lift my mail tray."

"I get this pain right here (pointing to a vertical line of pain running up the upper arm) whenever I move my shoulder."

"My shoulder has been sore for a long time. Yesterday, I tried to place my trailer on the trailer hitch when I felt and heard this loud pop."

"My shoulder used to hurt a lot every day. Two days ago, it stopped hurting. Now I have this big bruise near my elbow, and the muscle seems bigger."

Exam   Each patient should be examined for swelling and inflammation along the bicipital groove along with an assessment of the integrity of the tendon.

EXAM SUMMARY

> 1. Local tenderness in the bicipital groove
> 2. Pain is aggravated by flexion of the elbow, isometrically
> 3. A painful arc may be present (p. 13)
> 4. A bulge in the antecubital fossa (rupture)

(1) Local tenderness is present in the bicipital groove approximately 1″ below the anterolateral tip of the acromion. The bicipital groove can be identified by palpating the anterior humeral head while passively internally and externally rotating the arm. (2) Pain is aggravated by resisting elbow flexion isometrically. The patient describes a line of pain along the anterior humerus. (3) Pain may be aggravated by passively abducting the arm (the painful arc maneuver), because the long head tendon traverses between the humeral head and the undersurface of the acromion on its way to attach to the glenoid process. (4) Rupture of the tendon is usually manifested by a bulging, several inches above the antecubital fossa and a large ecchymosis present along the inner aspect of the distal arm. Strength of elbow flexion is usually preserved, because the short head and the brachioradialis tendons combine to make up 80% of the strength of elbow flexion.

X-Rays   X-rays of the shoulder are not always necessary. Plain films may demonstrate calcification in the bicipital groove; however, treatment decisions are based on clinical grounds rather than on the presence or absence of calcification.

Diagnosis   The diagnosis is suggested by a history of anterior humeral pain and by an exam showing local tenderness in the bicipital groove that is aggravated by resisted elbow flexion. A regional anesthetic block in the bicipital groove may be necessary to differentiate biceps tendinitis from referred pain from the rotator cuff tendons or pain arising from the glenohumeral joint.

Treatment   The goals of treatment are to reduce the inflammation and swelling in the tendon, to strengthen the biceps muscle and tendon, and to prevent rupture.

Step 1: Eliminate lifting.
> Restrict over-the-shoulder positions and reaching.
> Apply ice over the anterolateral shoulder.
> Suggest an NSAID (e.g., ibuprofen [Advil, Motrin]) for 3 to 4 weeks.
> Educate the patient. "If restrictions aren't followed, there is a 5 to 10% risk of rupture."

Step 2 (4 to 6 weeks): A local injection is given in the bicipital groove or in the subacromial bursa with D80 for patients younger than 50 years of age.
> Repeat the injection in 4 to 6 weeks if symptoms have not decreased by at least 50%.
> Combine the injection with a simple sling or shoulder immobilizer to provide maximum protection against rupture (see pp. 169 to 170).

Step 3 (2 to 3 months): Consider orthopedic consultation for persistent symptoms or if rupture has occurred.

Physical Therapy   Physical therapy plays a minor role in the treatment of bicipital tendinitis and bicipital tendon rupture.

PHYSICAL THERAPY SUMMARY

---

1. Ice
2. Phonophoresis
3. Weighted pendulum stretch exercises for uncomplicated bicipital tendinitis
4. Toning exercises for the short head biceps tendon and brachioradialis for bicipital tendon rupture

---

ACUTELY Ice, phonophoresis, and the weighted pendulum stretch exercises are used in the early treatment of bicipital tendinitis. *Ice* placed over the anterior humeral head provides temporary relief of pain. *Phonophoresis* over the anterior humeral head may provide relief of pain and swelling in thin patients. For an uncomplicated case of bicipital tendinitis, *weighted pendulum stretch exercises* are performed daily (see p. 145). Increasing the subacromial space can provide the long head tendon more freedom of motion.

Recovery/Rehabilitation Weighted pendulum stretch exercises are combined with isometric toning of the elbow flexors.

Weighted pendulum stretch exercises are continued through the recovery period. When these exercises are performed three times a week, the chance of recurrent tendinitis is reduced.

Three to four weeks after the acute pain has resolved, *isometric toning exercises of elbow flexion* are begun. These should be performed at 45 degrees of passive abduction of the shoulder to minimize the amount of friction in the bicipital groove. Daily toning exercises are particularly important when bicipital tendon rupture has occurred. Strengthening the short head of the biceps and brachioradialis just 15 to 20% will counteract the loss of strength from the rupture of the long head of the biceps.

INJECTION TECHNIQUE Local injection must be performed with caution, especially in patients over the age of 50 years. Prior to any injection, the patient must be advised of the risk of rupture. A subacromial injection is probably safer but unfortunately not as effective (p. 14).

Position: The patient is placed in a sitting position with the hands in the lap and asked to relax the shoulder and neck muscles.

Technique: The bicipital groove is identified just below the anterolateral tip of the acromion (with the examiner's fingers over the anterolateral humeral head, the groove will be palpable when the arm is passively rotated internally and then externally). An 1½" 25-gauge needle is passed down into the groove to the bone. Be sure to keep the bevel of the needle parallel to the fibers of the tendon. Inject only under light pressure. Approximately 2 to 3 ml of anesthetic is injected into the groove. The shoulder is re-examined. If the local tenderness and the pain from isometric testing of arm flexion is remarkably improved, 1 ml of D80 is injected in the same area.

Restrictions: Lifting is absolutely restricted for 1 month. Overhead reaching should be limited, because the long head of the biceps runs just under the subacromial bursa on its course to the glenoid labrum.

Prognosis A significant number of patients develop degenerative change in the tendon. Spontaneous rupture occurs in 10% of cases. Surprisingly, little functional disability results; the short head of the biceps and the brachioradialis provide 80% of the strength of elbow flexion. Rupture often cures the problem but leads to a minor deformity. For these reasons, surgical repair is not frequently suggested. Heavy laborers, violinists, and other patients who demand the utmost from their upper extremities should be referred for surgical consultation.

Elbow

LATERAL EPICONDYLITIS

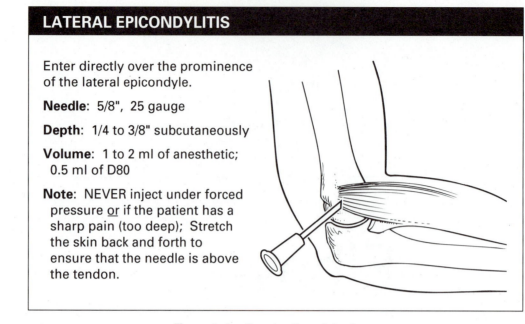

Enter directly over the prominence of the lateral epicondyle.

Needle: 5/8", 25 gauge

Depth: 1/4 to 3/8" subcutaneously

Volume: 1 to 2 ml of anesthetic; 0.5 ml of D80

Note: NEVER inject under forced pressure <u>or</u> if the patient has a sharp pain (too deep); Stretch the skin back and forth to ensure that the needle is above the tendon.

Figure 3–1. Tennis elbow injection.

Description   Lateral epicondylitis (tennis elbow) is an injury of the common extensor tendon at the lateral epicondyle of the humerus. Overuse of the wrist causes microtearing of the origin of the extensor carpi radialis and the extensor carpi ulnaris. Secondary inflammation develops at the epicondyle after this mechanical injury. The radiohumeral joint range of motion and function is unaffected.

Symptoms   The patient has elbow pain and weakness of the arm.

''The pain in my elbow has gotten so bad that I can't even lift my coffee cup.''

''After a couple of hours of using my screwdriver, my elbow starts to ache really badly.''

''I was pounding nails over the weekend, and ever since then my elbow has been aching.''

''Anytime I try to use my torque wrench, I get this sharp pain on the outside of my elbow.''

''You've got to do something, doc. I can't spike the volleyball anymore!''

Exam   Each patient should be examined for local irritation at the lateral epicondyle, along with the strength and integrity of the common extensor tendon mechanism.

EXAM SUMMARY

1. Local epicondylar tenderness
2. Pain aggravated by resisting wrist extension and radial deviation isometrically
3. Full range of motion of the elbow

(1) Local tenderness is most common over a dime-sized area at the lateral epicondyle. A few patients will have local tenderness between the radial head and the lateral epicondyle (the radial humeral bursa, an extension of the joint lining of the elbow).

(2) This lateral elbow pain is aggravated by resisting wrist extension and by radial deviation isometrically (the function of the extensor carpi radialis, which is the tendon most often involved). In more advanced cases, it may be aggravated by strong gripping. (3) The range of motion of the elbow is preserved. Loss of extension or flexion is almost always indicative of a primary elbow joint process.

X-Rays   X-rays of the elbow are not necessary. Routine films of the elbow are almost always normal and rarely influence treatment decisions.

Diagnosis   The diagnosis is based on the lateral epicondylar pain and on local tenderness aggravated by isometric wrist extension. Regional anesthetic block at the epicondyle confirms the diagnosis and helps to differentiate this local musculoskeletal pain from the referred pain of carpal tunnel syndrome, cervical radiculopathy, or rotator cuff tendinitis.

Treatment   The goals of treatment are to allow the common extensor tendon to reattach its origin to the lateral epicondylar process, to reduce the inflammation at the epicondyle, allowing the tendon to reattach, and to perform toning exercises of the forearm, helping to reduce the rate of recurrence.

Step 1: Limit lifting, hammering, and repetitive wrist and hand work.

Apply ice over the epicondyle.

Use a Velcro wrist splint (p. 172).

A nonsteroidal anti-inflammatory drug (NSAID) (e.g., ibuprofen [Advil, Motrin]) may be helpful.

Educate the patient, "You may feel the pain at the elbow, but it is the wrist and hand motions that have caused and aggravated it."

Step 2 (3 to 4 weeks): A short arm cast is used (p. 172) to replace the splint.

A long arm cast is necessary if supination and pronation of the forearm prominently affect the pain at the elbow.

Discontinue the NSAID.

Continue with application of ice.

Step 3 (6 to 8 weeks): A local injection of D80 is given if 3 weeks of casting has failed.

Repeat the injection in 4 to 6 weeks if symptoms have not been reduced by at least 50%.

Step 4 (6 to 10 weeks): Begin toning exercises (p. 149) after the pain has subsided.

Use a tennis elbow band (p. 171) to prevent a recurrence.

Gradually resume activities.

Demonstrate "palms-up lifting."

Consider an orthopedic referral for persistent symptoms, especially in the use of laborers and carpenters.

Physical Therapy   Physical therapy plays a minor role in the active treatment of the tendinitis of the common extensor origin and a vital role in its rehabilitation.

PHYSICAL THERAPY SUMMARY

1. Ice
2. Phonophoresis with a hydrocortisone gel
3. Isometric toning of gripping
4. Isometric toning of wrist extension

ACUTELY   *Ice* and *phonophoresis* using a hydrocortisone gel provide temporary relief of pain and swelling. Ice is routinely recommended and is particularly helpful for inflammatory flare reactions after local corticosteroid injection. Phonophoresis is used when inflammatory changes are prominent on physical exam. Both must be combined with immobilization to be effective.

RECOVERY/REHABILITATION Isometric exercises are used to restore the strength and tone of the extensor muscles. Three to 4 weeks after the symptoms and signs have resolved, *isometric toning exercises* are begun (p. 149). Initially, *grip exercises* using grip putty, a small compressible rubber ball, or an old tennis ball are performed daily in sets of 20, with each held for 5 seconds. The strength and endurance of the forearm flexor and extensor muscles are gradually built up. (When actively flexing the forearm muscles by gripping, the extensor muscles are activated as well.) These exercises are followed by *isometric toning exercises of wrist extension,* which are essential in preventing recurrent tendinitis. Each episode of epicondylitis weakens the common extensor mechanism. In order to overcome the loss of tensile strength, toning exercises need to be continued three times per week and combined with an ongoing limitation of lifting, torquing, and gripping.

Injection Technique The mechanical irritation that plays such a central role in the cause and aggravation of this tendinitis is best treated with wrist immobilization. Almost 70% of cases respond to splinting or casting. Those failing immobilization should be treated with local injection. Patients should be warned, however, that postinjection pain is frequent and that 30% will experience subcutaneous atrophy or discoloration at the injection site (this is a temporary effect in most cases; the skin and fat return to normal in 6 to 9 months).

Position: The patient is asked to lie down, to bend the elbow to 90 degrees, and to place the hand under the ipsilateral buttock.

Technique: The injection is placed at the prominence of the epicondyle, "just over" the tendon. The needle enters the skin over the center of the epicondyle and is advanced through the subcutaneous fat to the firm resistance of the tendon. A local anesthetic is placed just over the tendon. A painful reaction or firm pressure when injecting suggests that the needle is too deep and is under the tendon! The needle must be pulled back until the medicine either flows freely or the patient no longer feels discomfort. After local anesthetic block, with the needle left in place, a ½ ml of D80 is injected over a dime-sized area of the epicondyle by utilizing skin traction to move the needle. Again, if the needle is above the tendon, the needle will move back and forth with skin traction!

Restrictions: Repetitious lifting, hammering, gripping, and grasping are limited for 3 days. After recovery at 4 weeks, grip exercises are begun to strengthen the forearm muscles (p. 149). Additionally, a tennis elbow band can be used to prevent a recurrence. It serves to dampen the pressure coming back to the epicondyle from the wrist.

Prognosis Adequate immobilization is critical for proper healing. Unfortunately, at least 25% of patients suffer a recurrence due to poor reattachment or to degenerative change. Retreatment is often necessary. Surgery is offered for persistent cases—those with 30 to 40% impairment in function (e.g., decreased grip strength by 30 to 40%, reduced lifting ability by 30 to 40%). It is difficult to justify surgery for a 10 to 20% decrease in function. Successful surgery may only provide 90% of normal tensile strength! Extensor carpi radialis brevis débridement and repair can be combined with lateral epicondylectomy, or a simple common extensor origin release can be performed. Only 5% of cases would qualify for surgery under these criteria.

OLECRANON BURSITIS

Enter at the base of the bursa, securing the needle in the subcutaneous tissue; advance the needle into the center of the bursa.

Needle: 1 1/2", 18 gauge

Depth: 1/4 to 3/8"

Volume: 1 ml of anesthetic; 0.5 ml of K40

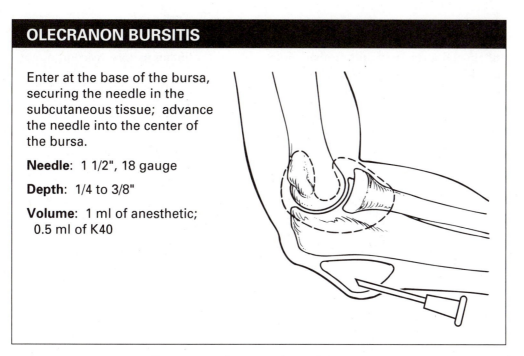

Figure 3–2. Olecranon bursa injection.

Description   Olecranon bursitis is an inflammation of the bursal sac, which is located between the olecranon process of the ulna and the overlying skin. It is a low-pressure bursa that is susceptible to swelling. Most cases are caused by repetitive trauma in the form of pressure—draftman's elbow. Five per cent are caused by gout, and 5% are caused by *Staphylococcus aureus* infection.

Symptoms   The patient has elbow pain and swelling just behind the elbow.

"Within 5 hours, I had this golf ball show up at the end of my elbow."

"I work as a draftsman. I slowly developed this swelling over my elbow."

"When I rub the skin over my elbow, I feel a bunch of little marbles."

"I've got this sack of fluid on my elbow."

"All of a sudden I developed this red, hot swollen area over my elbow."

Exam   Each patient should be examined for the degree of swelling and inflammation directly over the olecranon process.

EXAM SUMMARY

1. Swelling, redness, and heat over the olecranon process
2. Full range of motion of the elbow
3. A characteristic aspirate

(1) Cystic swelling, redness, or heat is present over the proximal 1" to 2" of the olecranon process. (2) The range of motion of the elbow should be unaffected. (3) The diagnosis is confirmed by aspiration of fluid from the bursal sac.

X-Rays   X-rays of the elbow are not necessary because they only show soft tissue swelling.

Diagnosis   The diagnosis is based on the laboratory evaluation of the bursal aspirate. The cell count, Gram stain, and crystal analysis will help to differentiate the inflammation of an acute traumatic bursitis from the inflammatory reaction of gout and infection! All bursae should be aspirated!

Treatment   The goals of treatment are to determine the cause of the swelling, to reduce swelling and inflammation, to encourage the walls of the bursa to reapproximate, and to prevent chronic bursitis.

Step 1: Aspirate the bursa for diagnostic studies: Gram stain and culture, uric acid crystals, and hematocrit.

A simple compression dressing for 24 to 36 hours (gauze and Elastoplast). Avoid direct pressure.

Use a neoprene pull-on elbow brace (p. 171).

Step 2 (1 to 2 days): Either give an antibiotic for the infection *(S. aureus)* or evaluate and treat for gout or give an intrabursal injection of K40 for the uncomplicated case of traumatic bursitis.

Continue the neoprene pull-on.

Step 3 (4 to 6 weeks): Repeat aspiration and local injection with K40 if there is persistent swelling and pain.

Educate the patient. "Ten to 20 per cent have persistently swollen or thickened sacs."

Step 4 (3 months): Consider an orthopedic consultation for a bursectomy if thickening has developed.

Physical Therapy   Physical therapy does not play a significant role in either the treatment or rehabilitation of olecranon bursitis.

Injection Technique   Aspiration or injection is the treatment of choice.

Position: The patient is asked to lie down. Place the patient's arm over the chest, and bend the elbow to 90 degrees (the sac will be tense in this position).

Technique: The base of the bursa is identified. Using a 25-gauge needle, 1 to 2 ml of local anesthetic is placed in the skin and subcutaneous tissue adjacent to the base of the bursa. A large-gauge needle is then used to remove all the fluid. The needle is passed into the center of the sac, and the bevel of the needle is rotated toward the olecranon. As much of the fluid as possible is aspirated. Studies are obtained. If the result of the stat Gram stain is negative, ½ ml of K40 is injected with the needle left in place.

Restrictions: A bulky pressure dressing is applied and is left in place for 24 to 36 hours. Direct pressure is avoided. A pull-on neoprene elbow brace is used for the next 30 days. The patient is advised to avoid any pressure over the olecranon and is warned about the possibility of a recurrence.

Prognosis   Fifty per cent of cases respond to simple aspiration. Another 30% respond to aspiration followed by K40 injection. Approximately one in five fails to resolve their symptoms and have persistent swelling or thickening of the sac. Surgical removal (bursectomy) can be performed on treatment failures, although this is more of a cosmetic surgery rather than a procedure to restore function. A chronically thickened bursal sac does not interfere with the function of the elbow. At most, the cobblestone-like thickening is irritating when pressure is applied to it.

CHAPTER 4

Wrist

DORSAL GANGLION

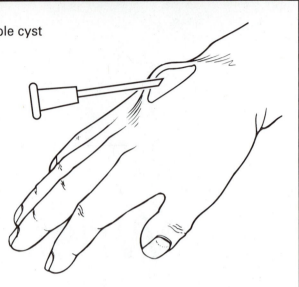

Enter at the base of the palpable cyst and parallel to the skin.

Needle: 1 1/2", 18 gauge

Depth: variable but rarely below 1/2"

Volume: 1/2 ml of local anesthetic, skin and subcutaneously

Note: a 10 ml syringe is necessary to obtain enough vacuum pressure; follow the puncture and aspiration with manual pressure.

Figure 4–1.   Ganglion aspiration.

Description   A dorsal ganglion is an abnormal accumulation of synovial or teno-synovial fluid. Subtle abnormalities in the wrist or the extensor tendon sheath cause an overproduction of fluid that leaks into the subcutaneous tissue. A cyst wall forms around the irritating fluid. Other names for this common condition include Bible cyst, wrist cyst, or dorsal tendon cyst.

Symptoms   The patient has a painless lump at the wrist.

''I noticed this swelling over my wrist. My brothers have all died of cancer, and I was very worried about it.''

''I developed this really ugly swelling over the back of my hand. I want it taken off.''

''I type all day long. Over the last several months I have noticed this lump on the back of my hand.''

''I've had this bump on the back of my wrist for years, but it recently has grown bigger.''

Exam   The characteristics (e.g., size, mobility, and compressibility) of the cyst are evaluated along with an assessment of the wrist joint and the function of the dorsal tendons that cross the wrist.

EXAM SUMMARY

1. A highly mobile, fluctuant cyst overlying the wrist
2. Minimal tenderness
3. Wrist motion is normal in most cases
4. A characteristic aspirate

(1) A 1- to 2-cm highly mobile, fluctuant to tense cyst is palpable in the subcutaneous tissue. It should not be grossly adherent to the underlying tissue. (2) Tenderness is minimal unless the cyst is pressing against one of the cutaneous nerves. (3) Wrist

motion is painless and full, unless there is underlying carpal or radiocarpal arthritis. (4) The diagnosis is confirmed by aspirating the thick, highly viscous, nearly colorless fluid from the cyst (the consistency of Karo syrup).

X-Rays   X-rays of the wrist are not necessary for the diagnosis because they are normal unless there is concurrent carpal or radiocarpal arthritis.

Diagnosis   Aspiration of the characteristic nonbloody aspirate is diagnostic.

Treatment   The goals of treatment are to reassure the patient that this is not a serious problem, to drain the abnormal accumulation of lubricating fluid, and to prevent a recurrence by strengthening the wrist and by advising on improved ergonomics.

Step 1: Observe the cyst, which may involute with time.
　　　　Educate the patient. "This may resolve spontaneously."
　　　　Do a simple aspiration.
　　　　Limit wrist motions, especially repetitious use.
　　　　Use a Velcro wrist brace (p. 172).

Step 2 (8 to 10 weeks): Repeat aspiration and inject with K40.
　　　　Continue the wrist brace.

Step 3 (12 weeks or longer): Consider a repeat injection with K40 (if smaller).
　　　　Perform gripping and wrist-toning exercises (p. 149).
　　　　Consider an orthopedic consultation for removal.
　　　　Educate the patient, "Some cases may recur even after surgical removal, depending on whether you continue to produce too much lubricating fluid."

Physical Therapy   The role of physical therapy is limited in the treatment and prevention of ganglia. Wrist-strengthening exercises are indicated if there is clinical evidence of underlying radiocarpal arthritis. Generally, isometric toning exercises are performed to strengthen wrist extension and flexion for patients who work heavily with their hands.

Injection Technique   Aspiration or injection is the treatment of choice for ganglions that do not resolve on their own; however, the cyst must be at least 1 cm in diameter in order to aspirate easily. First occurrences are treated with simple aspiration. Recurrences can be treated with aspiration followed by injection with a corticosteroid.

Position: To facilitate aspiration, the wrist is flexed to 45 degrees and is held in place with a towel rolled up underneath it.

Technique: Anesthesia is placed in the skin and at the base of the ganglion, using a 25-gauge needle. An 18-gauge needle attached to a 10-ml syringe is advanced through the subcutaneous tissue and into the cyst. When the needle is centered in the cyst, the bevel is rotated 180 degrees. All of the highly viscous fluid is removed. Manual pressure is applied to either side of the cyst to assist in removal of the fluid. Without moving the needle, ½ ml of K40 is injected into the center of the cyst. Light pressure is applied immediately after injection to prevent escape of the steroid into the subcutaneous tissue.

Restrictions: Wrist motion is restricted for 3 days. Repetitious wrist motion is limited for the next 30 days. Recurrent cases may benefit from concurrent Velcro bracing.

Prognosis   Ganglions recur despite medical or surgical treatment. A recurrence depends more on the underlying cause of the overproduced synovial fluid rather than on the type of treatment. Simple excision is the surgical treatment of choice.

DE QUERVAIN TENOSYNOVITIS

Enter 3/8" distal to the radial styloid and angle at 45 degrees down to the bone.

Needle: 5/8", 25 gauge

Depth: 3/8", flush against the styloid tip

Volume: 2 ml of anesthetic; 0.5 ml of D80

Note: the tenosynovial sac should distend and form a bubble.

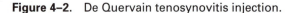

Figure 4–2. De Quervain tenosynovitis injection.

Description De Quervain tenosynovitis is an inflammation of the extensor and abductor tendons of the thumb. Overuse or unaccustomed use in the form of repetitive gripping and grasping leads to friction irritation of the snuffbox tendons as they cross the distal radial styloid. If left untreated, this friction-induced tenosynovitis can progress to fibrosis of the tenosynovial sac and to loss of flexibility of the thumb in flexion. The latter condition is referred to as stenosing tenosynovitis.

Symptoms The patient has wrist pain and difficulties with gripping.

"I can't grip anymore."

"Every time I try to pick up my baby, I get this sharp pain in my wrist."

"I have had this sharp pain over my wrist (pointing to the end of the radius) every since I had this needle stuck in my vein."

"It's very sore right here (pointing to the end of the radius), and it has begun to swell."

"My bone is getting bigger (pointing to the radial styloid of the radius)."

Exam Each patient should be examined for inflammation of the extensor pollicis longus, extensor pollicis brevis, and abductor pollicis longus along with an assessment of the degree of fibrosis in the tenosynovial sac.

EXAM SUMMARY

1. Local tenderness at the tip of the radial styloid
2. Pain aggravated by isometric thumb extension or abduction
3. A positive result on the Finklestein test (stretching the thumb tendons)
4. A distensible tenosynovial sac

(1) Local tenderness is present at the tip of the radial styloid, adjacent to the abductor pollicis longus tendon. (2) Pain is aggravated by resisting thumb extension and abduction isometrically. (Thumb abduction is moving the thumb perpendicular to the palm.) (3) Pain is aggravated by stretching the thumb tendons over the radial styloid in thumb flexion (the Finklestein maneuver). This maneuver is so painful that the patient often responds by lifting the shoulder to prevent the examiner from stretching the tendon! (4) The degree of fibrosis is determined by the distensibility of

the tenosynovial sac and by the flexibility of the thumb tendons in flexion. Thumb flexion should be compared side to side. Normally, the tenosynovial sac should distend readily with 2 to 3 ml of local anesthetic.

X-Rays   X-rays of the wrist and thumb are not necessary. Plain films of the wrist and thumb are normal, and calcification of these tendons does not occur.

Diagnosis   The diagnosis is suggested by a history of wrist pain and an exam showing local radial styloid tenderness aggravated by resisting thumb extension. The diagnosis is confirmed by a regional anesthetic block placed in the tenosynovial sac. Effective relief of signs and symptoms excludes carpometacarpal arthritis and radiocarpal arthritis. A distensible tenosynovial sac effectively rules out stenosing tenosynovitis.

Treatment   The goals of treatment are to reduce the inflammation in the tenosynovial sac, to prevent adhesions from forming, and to prevent recurrent tendinitis (by tendon stretch exercises and by altering lifting and grasping).

Step 1: Rest and restrict thumb gripping and grasping.
Apply ice at the radial styloid.
Buddy tape the thumb to the base of the first finger (p. 176); apply a dorsal hood splint (p. 173); or apply a Velcro thumb spica splint (p. 174).

Step 2 (4 to 6 weeks): Give a local injection with D80.
Repeat the injection at 4 to 6 weeks if the symptoms are not reduced by 50%.
Severe cases that require a second injection can be treated with either a dorsal hood splint or a short-arm cast with a thumb spica (p. 175).

Step 3 (10 to 12 weeks): Apply gentle stretch exercises of the thumb into the palm if the patient has improved (p. 150).
Consider surgical release for persistent symptoms.

Physical Therapy   Physical therapy has a minor role in the treatment of De Quervain tenosynovitis.

PHYSICAL THERAPY SUMMARY

1. Ice
2. Phonophoresis
3. Gentle stretch exercises in flexion (prevention)

ACUTELY   Ice and phonophoresis are used in the treatment of active tenosynovitis. *Ice* applied to the radial styloid can effectively reduce local pain and swelling. *Phonophoresis* with a hydrocortisone gel may be helpful in minor cases but cannot take the place of a local corticosteroid injection in persistent or chronic cases.

RECOVERY/REHABILITATION   Stretching exercises are used to prevent a recurrence. After the signs of symptoms of active tenosynovitis have resolved (3 to 4 weeks), gentle *passive stretching* of the extensor tendons into the palm is recommended. Sets of 20 stretches, each held 5 seconds, are performed daily (p. 150). These are especially important for cases complicated by stenosis.

Injection Technique   Local injection with D80 is the preferred treatment when simple rest and immobilization fail to resolve the problem in 6 weeks.

Position: The wrist is turned on its side, radial side up. The wrist joint is kept in a neutral position.

Technique: The tip of the radial styloid and the snuffbox tendons are identified. A 25-gauge needle enters just over the tip of the radial styloid, halfway between the abductor pollicis longus and the extensor pollicis longus tendons.

The needle is advanced at a 45-degree angle down to the hard resistance of the radial styloid (painful!). Local anesthetic is placed flush against the bone. A bubble should form, ensuring placement in the tenosynovial sac. A poorly distensible sac may indicate a chronic stenosis of the tendons (i.e., adhesions). With the needle left in place (only one puncture of the tenosynovial sac), 1/2 ml of D80 is injected.

Restrictions: Splinting can be continued for the first few days to ensure that the steroid remains properly positioned. Gripping and grasping are restricted for 30 days.

Prognosis   A local injection is highly successful. One or two injections will be successful in 90% of cases. Thirty per cent will require reinjection at 1 year. Ten per cent of cases fail to respond to this treatment and can be considered for surgery. Release of the retinaculum at the wrist (tenovaginotomy of the first dorsal compartment) is successful in 90% of cases.

CARPOMETACARPAL OSTEOARTHRITIS

Enter 3/8" proximal to the base of the metacarpal and between the snuffbox tendons.

Needle: 5/8", 25 gauge

Depth: 5/8", flush against the trapezium bone

Volume: 1 to 2 ml of anesthetic; 0.5 ml D80 or K40

Note: apply moderate pressure.

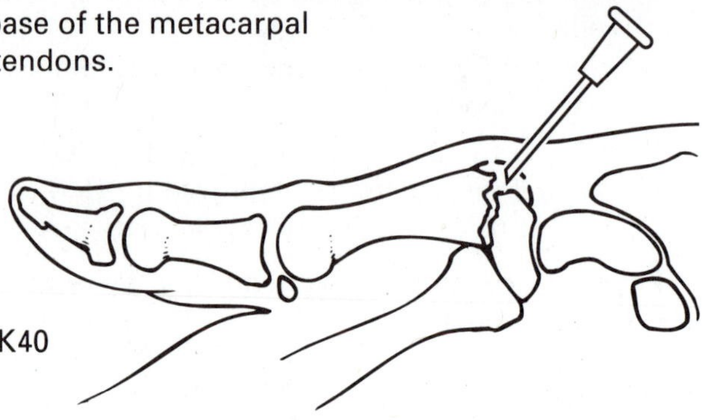

Figure 4–3.   Thumb arthritis injection.

Description   Carpometacarpal (CMC) joint arthritis is a very common manifestation of osteoarthritis. Repetitive gripping, repetitive grasping, and excessive contact with vibration tools in a susceptible patient (positive family history) leads to wear and tear of the bones at the base of the thumb. Over many years, bony enlargement, loss of range of motion, and progressive subluxation occur.

Symptoms   The patient has pain, swelling, or enlargement at the base of the thumb.

"I've had to stop crocheting and knitting because of the constant pain in my thumbs."

"My thumbs are starting to look like the arthritis my grandmother had."

"Every time I lift my coffee cup, I get this terribly sharp pain in the base of my thumb."

"I can't move my thumbs very much without pain."

"It looks like the bones in my thumb are getting bigger."

Exam   Each patient should be examined for swelling and inflammation at the base of the thumb, along with the degree of subluxation of the metacarpal bone and loss of range of motion of the joint.

EXAM SUMMARY

> **1.** Compression tenderness across the joint
> **2.** Crepitation of the joint in circumduction
> **3.** Pain aggravated at the extremes of thumb motion
> **4.** Bony deformity and or subluxation (the shelf sign)
> **5.** Atrophy of the thenar muscles
---

(1) Tenderness is present over the swollen base of the thumb and is best demonstrated by compressing the joint in the anteroposterior plane. Pressure applied from the snuffbox is usually much less painful. (2) Crepitation is palpable when forcibly rotating the metacarpal against the trapezium (the mortar and pestle sign). (3) Pain is often aggravated when passively stretching the joint at the extremes of extension and flexion. (4) As the condition progresses, bone deformity and subluxation contribute to the enlargement of the base of the thumb. Progressive subluxation creates an abnormality referred to as the shelf sign. (The smooth contours of the distal radius and thumb are replaced by a bony protuberance of the metacarpal.) (5) End-stage disease often shows atrophy of the thenar muscles.

X-Rays   X-rays of the wrist and thumb are necessary. Symptomatic cases will have abnormal plain films of the thumb. Variable degrees of bony sclerosis, asymmetric joint narrowing, spur formation, and radial side subluxation can be seen at the trapezial-metacarpal articulation.

Diagnosis   The diagnosis is based on the clinical findings of local joint tenderness, joint crepitation, and painful motion of the joint coupled with the characteristic abnormalities on plain films of the thumb. X-rays are often used to gauge the severity of the condition and to predict the need for surgery. A regional anesthetic block is occasionally necessary to differentiate de Quervain tenosynovitis from symptomatic CMC arthritis.

Treatment   The goals of treatment are to palliate symptoms, to reduce swelling and inflammation (allowing the joint to articulate more properly), and to assess the need for surgery.

Step 1: X-ray the wrist and thumb.
> Rest and restrict gripping and grasping.
> Use oversize tools, grips, and other occupation adjustments.
> Overlap taping of the joint and the radial side of the wrist (p. 175) or a dorsal hood splint (p. 173) or a thumb spica Velcro splint (p. 174).
> A 4-week course of a nonsteroidal anti-inflammatory drug (NSAID) (e.g., ibuprofen [Advil, Motrin]).

Step 2 (4 to 6 weeks): Give a local injection with D80.
> Repeat the injection at 4 to 6 weeks if symptoms have not decreased by 50%.

Step 3 (3 months): Use a thumb spica cast (p. 175) with or without a local injection.

Step 4 (4 to 6 months): Do isometric toning exercises of the thumb flexors and extensors (if improved).
> Consult with a hand surgeon for implant arthroplasty or tendon graft interposition, depending on the patient's age.

Physical Therapy   Physical therapy does not have a significant role in the treatment of CMC osteoarthritis. The focus of therapy is on restricted use, bracing, and anti-inflammatory treatments. If significant loss of muscle tone has occurred, isometric toning of flexion, extension, abduction, and adduction are recommended. Preferential toning of extension (almost always weaker than flexion) may reduce the tendency of the joint to sublux.

Injection Technique   Local injection is effective for this arthritic condition; however, the response is unpredictable. Most patients experience relief for months, whereas others fail to respond. For patients younger than 55 years of age, an injection can provide sufficient relief prior to definitive surgery.

Position: The wrist is turned on its side, radial side up. The wrist joint is kept in a neutral position.

Technique: The base of the thumb is identified. The skin is entered just proximal to the head of the metacarpal, halfway between the extensor pollicis longus and the abductor pollicis longus tendons. The needle is positioned at a 45-degree angle and is gently passed down to the trapezium bone. The needle may need to be redirected if bone is encountered at a superficial level, approximately ⅜″. Firm but not hard pressure may be required when injecting.

Restrictions: Grasping and pinching are restricted for 30 days. Lighter gripping of the pen, padding of hand tools, avoidance of vibratory tools, and use of oversized golf grips are suggested. Isometric exercises to strengthen thumb extension and abduction may improve long-term results.

Prognosis   Local injection is highly successful in the short term in most patients. A single injection can provide symptomatic relief and improved function, especially when swelling predominates. When conservative care fails to control symptoms, surgery is offered. Replacement of the trapezium is usually reserved for patients older than 65 years of age (implant arthroplasty). Tendon graft arthroplasty (interposition of the flexor carpi radialis tendon between the bones of the joint) is the treatment offered to patients younger than 65 years of age.

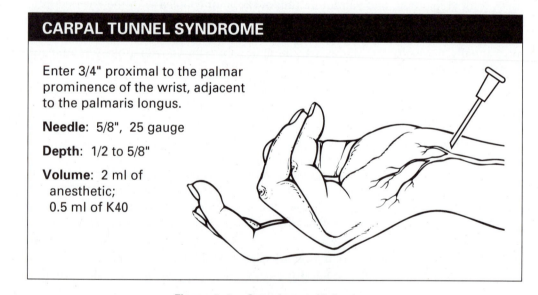

CARPAL TUNNEL SYNDROME

Enter 3/4" proximal to the palmar prominence of the wrist, adjacent to the palmaris longus.

Needle: 5/8", 25 gauge

Depth: 1/2 to 5/8"

Volume: 2 ml of anesthetic; 0.5 ml of K40

Figure 4–4.   Carpal tunnel injection.

Description   Carpal tunnel syndrome (CTS) is a compression neuropathy of the median nerve. Compression most commonly occurs at the transverse carpal ligament at the wrist but may also occur in the proximal forearm at the pronator teres muscle or in the distal forearm (rarely) following trauma. Traditionally and anatomically, the term CTS is used to refer to the former and median neuropathy for any condition that causes median nerve symptoms. The stage of the condition (from sensory loss to motor loss to motor loss with atrophy) correlates directly with the degree of compression and the chronicity of the symptoms. Most cases present at an early stage with intermittent sensory symptoms.

Symptoms   The patient has a loss of sensation in the tips of the first three digits, forearm and wrist pain, or weakness of grip.

''My thumb and first two fingers go to sleep at night.''

''After I've typed all day, I get these shooting pains up and down my arm.''

''My hand keeps going numb.''

''After long bike rides, my fingers go to sleep.''

''My hand feels dead. I've started to drop things.''

Exam   Each patient should have median nerve function tested by examining the sensation of the first three digits and the strength of thumb opposition along with an assessment of nerve irritability, either at the volar wrist or in the forearm.

EXAM SUMMARY

---

1. Sensory loss in the first three fingers
2. Loss of thumb opposition
3. Tinel sign and Phalen sign
4. Pressure over the pronator teres
5. Median nerve block

Depending on the time of day, the amount of use, and the daily variation of symptoms, the examination of the median nerve may be totally normal despite a clinically significant problem. (1) Two-point discrimination, light touch, and pain sensation may be decreased at the fingertips of the first three digits. (2) The strength of thumb opposition may be decreased. This is best performed by asking the patient to hold the thumb and fifth finger together. (3) Tinel sign and Phalen sign are performed at the wrist to test nerve irritability. Tinel sign should be performed with vigorous tapping over the transverse carpal ligament with the wrist held in extension. Phalen sign should be held for 30 to 60 seconds. (4) If these results are negative, then compression in the forearm should be performed. Pressure is applied 1″ to 2″ distal to the antecubital fossa. (5) Further confirmation of the diagnosis can be made by median nerve block at the wrist or short-term response to corticosteroid injection. Note that median nerve distribution varies from one patient to another. Most patients experience paresthesia in the first three digits; however, a few patients may experience symptoms in the second and third fingers with little involvement of the thumb or even in the radial side of the fourth digit.

Special Testing   No characteristic radiographic changes occur with CTS. X-rays of the wrist are not necessary unless there is clinical evidence of an underlying carpal or radiocarpal arthritis. Nerve conduction velocity (NCV) testing is the test of choice. The result of an NCV will be positive in approximately 70% of cases. Note that a negative result on an NCV does *not* totally exclude the presence of median nerve compression.

Diagnosis   In advanced cases (e.g., prolonged symptoms, motor involvement), the NCV test is the diagnostic test of choice and has high predictive value; however, patients with intermittent symptoms or mild sensory symptoms present a diagnostic dilemma. The result of the NCV is often normal in these patients. When the diagnosis is suspected on clinical grounds (e.g., characteristic pain pattern, Tinel sign, Phalen sign), a regional anesthetic block plus a corticosteroid injection should be considered. Almost 90% of patients experience relief from this procedure, helping to confirm the clinical suspicion of CTS.

Treatment   The goals of treatment are to reduce pressure over the nerve, to reduce concurrent flexor tenosynovitis, and to prevent a recurrence by improved use and ergonomics.

Step 1: Evaluate the stage of the condition and the underlying cause (by clinical testing or NCV).

Treat the underlying cause using diuretics or anti-inflammatory medications for rheumatoid arthritis or levothyroxine for hypothyroidism.

Reduce repetitive wrist motion.

Use antivibration padded gloves (Sorbothane).

Reposition the wrist at the keyboard, assembly line, and so forth.

Use a Velcro wrist splint at night (p. 172).

Step 2 (2 to 4 weeks): Re-evaluate the stage of the condition.

All patients should have an NCV for persistent symptoms and especially if motor symptoms are present.

Give a local injection of the tunnel with K40 (for sensory symptoms only!).

Use a Velcro wrist splint during the day and at night.

Repeat the injection in 4 to 6 weeks if symptoms have not been reduced by 50%.

Step 3 (8 to 10 weeks): Stretch exercises for the flexor tendons are begun if symptoms have improved (p. 150).

Rediscuss ergonomics and proper use.

Request a surgical consultation if motor symptoms have developed or symptoms have failed to improve.

Physical Therapy   Although surgical release is still the mainstay of treatment, more and more emphasis has been placed on the role of physical therapy in the treatment of CTS. Ergonomic adjustments in position and use can have a tremendous impact on the active treatment and rehabilitation of the condition. The anatomic positions of the hand and wrist are always suggested and preferred. In addition, stretch exercises of the flexor tendons of the hand may reduce the overall irritation of the median nerve (p. 150). These stretch exercises are especially helpful when combined with local corticosteroid injection.

Injection Technique   Local injection as a definitive treatment should be limited to patients with sensory symptoms only. Advanced cases should be offered surgery.

Position: The volar wrist is flexed to 45 degrees and is held in place with a towel rolled up underneath it.

Technique: The injection is placed under the transverse carpal ligament. The needle is inserted ½″ to ¾″ proximal to the palmar prominence of the wrist adjacent to the palmaris longus tendon. The needle is advanced at a 45-degree angle down to and through the ligament. Often a pop or giving way is felt when the needle passes through the ligament. Firm pressure is often necessary to push through the ligament. The medications should flow in with minimal pressure. If the patient experiences too much medial nerve irritation, the needle is withdrawn 1 or 2 mm.

Restrictions: Restriction of wrist motion is strictly adhered to for the next 3 days. The wrist splint is used for the next 30 days. Flexor tendon stretching should begin after 4 weeks.

Prognosis   Medical therapy provides long-term control of symptoms in less than half of patients. A local injection is highly effective in the short term (months), but only 25% have long-term benefit over years. Symptoms often persist because of secondary factors, especially repetitive wrist and hand use, uncontrollable factors on the job, and unavoidable vibration. Surgery is indicated for persistent or slowly progressive nerve dysfunction or motor loss (e.g., loss of grip, specific loss of thumb opposition). Surgical release of the transverse carpal ligament is successful in 90% of cases. Ten per cent of cases fail to improve due to nerve damage, postoperative neuritis, or recurrent compression due to scar tissue formation.

Hand

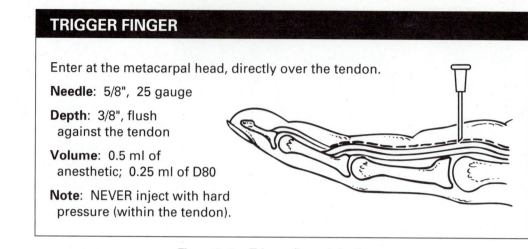

Figure 5–1. Trigger finger injection.

Description Trigger finger is an inflammation of the flexor tendons of the finger as they cross the metacarpophalangeal (MCP) head in the palm. Repetitive gripping and grasping or pressure over the palm causes swelling and inflammation of the tendon and the tendon sheath (tenosynovitis). As the swelling increases, the two flexor tendons lose their smooth motion under the A1 pulley, and the finger begins to catch or lock (triggering).

Symptoms The patient complains either of a painful finger or of loss of smooth motion of the finger when gripping or pinching.

"My finger keeps catching."

"I wake up in the morning and my finger is locked."

"My finger has started to tie up again."

"The dumb thing locks down."

"I had to stop knitting because my finger hurts all the time."

"If I use scissors or fingernail clippers, I get this sharp pain in my finger (pointing to the base of the finger in the palm)."

"I just thought that this was arthritis! I ignored the pain for the longest time. I didn't know that it could be treated."

Exam Each patient should be examined for active tenosynovitis of the flexor tendons of the finger along with the degree of mechanical locking.

EXAM SUMMARY

1. Local tenderness at the MCP head
2. Pain with stretch in extension
3. Pain with isometric flexion
4. Mechanical locking

(1) Local tenderness is present at the base of the digit directly over the tendon at the metacarpal head. Ten per cent of cases will also have subtle palpable swelling. (2) Pain is aggravated by stretching the tendon in extension or (3) by resisting the action of flexion isometrically. (4) Clicking or locking with active flexion may or may not be present, depending on the time of day or how long the patient has had the symptoms.

X-Rays   X-rays of the hand are not necessary. Calcification of the tendon does not occur.

Diagnosis   The diagnosis is based on a history of locking and on an exam showing three of the four main signs (e.g., locking, local tenderness at the MCP head, painful stretching in extension, or isometrically resisted flexion). A regional anesthetic block is rarely necessary to make the diagnosis, except in the case of tenosynovitis complicating an early Dupuytren contracture.

Treatment   The goals of treatment are to reduce the swelling and inflammation in the flexor tendon sheath, to allow smoother movement of the tendon under the A1 pulley, and to perform stretch exercises in extension to reduce the possibility of a recurrence.

Step 1: Restrict gripping and pinching.
    Buddy tape to the adjacent finger (p. 176).
    Apply ice over the metacarpal head.
    Apply a metal finger splint (p. 177).
    Use antivibration padded gloves (Sorbothane).
    Nonsteroidal anti-inflammatory drugs (NSAIDs) do not help.
Step 2 (4 to 6 weeks): Give a local injection with D80.
    Repeat the injection at 6 weeks if symptoms are not relieved by at least 50%.
Step 3 (10 to 12 weeks): Use padded or oversized tools.
    Lessen the tension when gripping or pinching.
    Recommend gentle stretch exercises in extension of the fingers (p. 150).
    Consider surgical release if symptoms are not relieved by two injections.

Physical Therapy   Physical therapy plays a minor role in the overall management of trigger finger. Stretching exercises in extension are used to prevent recurrent tenosynovitis and to rehabilitate the tendons in the postoperative recovery period. Sets of 20 gentle stretches are performed daily to maintain flexor tendon mobility and to reduce the contracture over the MCP head. Physical therapy is not appropriate for active tenosynovitis.

Injection Technique   A local injection is the treatment of choice. If simple immobilization fails after 4 to 6 weeks, an injection should be performed.

Position: The hand is placed flat on the exam table with the palm up and the fingers outstretched.

Technique: The distal head of the metacarpal bone is identified. The needle enters in the midline, just over the metacarpal head, and is passed down vertically to the firm resistance of the tendon. The tendon has a rubbery consistency. The anesthetic and corticosteroid are injected with the needle held flush against the tendon. A painful reaction suggests that the injection is too deep and is likely to be in the tendon!

Restrictions: Avoid gripping and grasping for 3 days. Splinting is not necessary.

Prognosis   A local injection with D80 is highly effective. Two thirds of cases require only one injection for long-term benefit. One quarter of cases require reinjection within 1 year. Ten per cent will fail medical therapy and require surgical release. This outpatient surgery is safe and effective. The fascial tissue over the tendon at the MCP head is sharply dissected. Recovery may take 3 to 4 weeks.

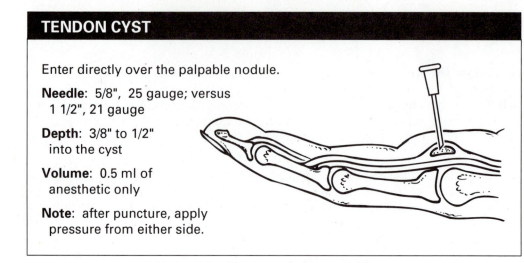

TENDON CYST

Enter directly over the palpable nodule.

Needle: 5/8", 25 gauge; versus
1 1/2", 21 gauge

Depth: 3/8" to 1/2"
into the cyst

Volume: 0.5 ml of
anesthetic only

Note: after puncture, apply
pressure from either side.

Figure 5–2.   Tendon cyst decompression.

Description   A tendon cyst is an abnormal collection of tenosynovial fluid, either within the tendon or adjacent to it. Direct, nonpenetrating trauma subtly damages the tendon or tendon sheath, causing a nodule to form. Despite its size (3 to 5 mm in diameter), the nodule rarely interferes with the function of the tendons or the adjacent MCP joint.

Symptoms   The patient complains of a lump in the palm of the hand, which is mildly tender.

"I have this small knot right here (pointing to the base of the finger in the palm)."

"Feel this thing, kind of like a little marble or B.B."

"When I use my little scissors and place pressure over my finger, I get a sharp pain."

"My doctor told me that I have a cyst in my tendon, but I'm not so sure that I believe him."

"Ever since I hit the countertop with my hand, I've felt this lump in my palm (pointing to the base of the finger)."

"I'm a professional percussionist. My favorite instrument is the tambourine. About four weeks ago, I noticed a pain along my fourth finger every time I tried to hold on to my tambourine. There's a small lump there now."

Exam   The location and size of the nodule, relative to the position of the tendon and metacarpal head, are assessed.

EXAM SUMMARY

1. A smooth, firm nodule 3 to 5 mm in diameter that is palpable in the palm
2. Very mild tenderness
3. Absence of mechanical locking, triggering, etc.

(1) A firm nodule is palpable in the palm adjacent to the distal metacarpal head. If the nodule is inside the tendon, passive motion of the finger in flexion and extension will cause it to move. If the nodule is adjacent to the tendon, the nodule is less likely to move directly with passive motion of the tendon. (2) Mild tenderness may be present over the nodule. (3) The flexor tendons are free of mechanical catching or

locking (i.e., the MCP and proximal interphalangeal [PIP] joints should have full, smooth flexion and extension).

X-Rays X-rays of the hand are not necessary. Calcification of the cyst and underlying bony changes do not occur.

Diagnosis A presumptive diagnosis is based on the size and location of the nodule in the palm. A simple puncture with decompression confirms the diagnosis. Those that do not decompress with a simple puncture may need to be confirmed surgically.

Treatment The goal of treatment is to decompress the abnormal accumulation of fluid inside the flexor tendon.

Step 1: Observe, because the nodule may resolve spontaneously.

Step 2 (4 to 8 weeks): Perform a simple puncture and decompression. Repeat the procedure if the cyst recurs.
   Reduce gripping and grasping tension; use padded tools or wear padded antivibration gloves.

Step 3 (months): Consider surgical decompression for persistent or symptomatic cysts.

Physical Therapy Physical therapy does not have a significant role in the treatment of tendon cysts.

Injection Technique Simple puncture is the treatment of choice.

Position: The hand is placed on the exam table with the palm up and the fingers outstretched.

Technique: The nodule is identified and held firmly with one finger above and one finger below the tendon. The needle is centered over the nodule and is passed vertically into the cyst at least twice. Aspiration is usually unsuccessful. Manual pressure using the barrel of a syringe in a "rolling fashion" or with the examiner's fingers will decompress most nodules. Repeat the procedure with a 21-gauge needle if the nodule is not reduced in size.

Restrictions: Reduce or adjust the pressure of pinching, gripping, and grasping.

Prognosis A simple puncture is highly effective. Surgical excision is indicated if the nodule persists and hand function is interfered with. Surgery for cosmetic results is to be discouraged. Postoperative scarring may limit finger mobility.

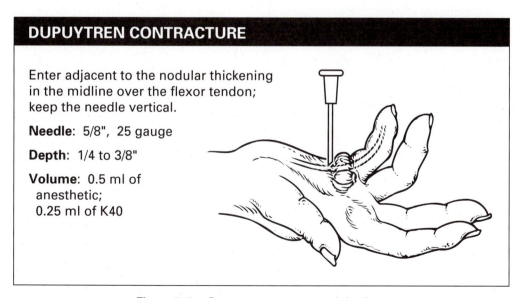

DUPUYTREN CONTRACTURE

Enter adjacent to the nodular thickening in the midline over the flexor tendon; keep the needle vertical.

Needle: 5/8", 25 gauge

Depth: 1/4 to 3/8"

Volume: 0.5 ml of anesthetic; 0.25 ml of K40

Figure 5–3. Dupuytren contracture injection.

Description   Dupuytren contracture is a progressive fibrosis of the palmar fascia. Tissue thickening envelopes the flexor tendons—typically the fourth and fifth tendons—and leads to the gradual contracture of the fingers into the palm. The majority of cases are idiopathic, although the occurrence is statistically higher in Scandinavians and in patients with advanced liver disease.

Symptoms   The patient complains of finger stiffness and loss of motion of the affected finger or thickening of the palm.

"I can't straighten my ring and little fingers."

"My fingers have slowly drawn down into my hand."

"I can't hold my hammer and small tools anymore. I can't open my hand enough."

"I've got these knots in my palm."

"My fingers won't straighten."

Exam   Each patient should be examined for the extent and location of the palmar fibrosis along with the impairment of flexion and extension in the affected fingers (i.e., the degree of flexion contracture of the fingers).

EXAM SUMMARY

> **1.** Painless palmar nodules
> **2.** Fixed flexion contracture of the affected fingers (usually the fourth and fifth)
> **3.** Inflammation notably absent

(1) Discrete nodules along the course of the flexor tendons are visible and palpable. The tendons of the fourth and fifth fingers are most frequently involved. (2) The flexibility of the MCP and PIP joints is reduced, leading to fixed flexion contractures (loss of full extension). (3) Signs of active inflammation are notably absent in most cases. Specifically, local tenderness, swelling, and pain with passive flexion and extension are absent unless a concurrent tenosynovitis is present (rare).

X-Rays   Plain films of the hand are not necessary. Calcification of the tendon does not occur.

Diagnosis   The diagnosis is based on the history of painless stiffness of the fingers and on the characteristic physical findings of peritendinous thickening and flexor tendon deformity. Note that on rare occasions, Dupuytren contracture can be painful. In the early stages, tenosynovitis can be present.

Treatment   The goals of treatment are to educate the patient regarding its slowly progressive nature over a period of years, to maintain the flexibility of the flexor tendons with stretch exercises, and to evaluate the need for surgery when significant functional loss has occurred.

Step 1: Educate the patient, "The process slowly worsens over many years."
    Heat the hand and massage the tendons with a heavy-based lanolin cream.
    Gently stretch the tendons in extension (p. 150).

Step 2 (months to years): If the pain of tenosynovitis occurs, a local injection with K40 can be tried.

Step 3 (years): Consider surgical release if the contracture progresses and interferes with function.
    Educate the patient, "Surgery will not cure the problem, only improve function temporarily."

Physical Therapy Physical therapy is the main form of treatment for early Dupuytren contracture (prior to surgical release).

PHYSICAL THERAPY SUMMARY

> **1.** Heat the hand
> **2.** Palm massage with a thick lanolin cream
> **3.** Gentle stretch exercises in extension

The hand is *heated* in warm water for 10 minutes. The flexor tendons of the affected fingers are *massaged* with a heavy-based lanolin cream. Sets of 20 gentle *stretch exercises in extension* are performed daily. Heavy gripping and grasping are altered.

Injection Technique For most patients, this problem is treated with observation and physical therapy. As the condition progresses and the contracture worsens, the principal therapy is surgery. A local injection is infrequently used unless tenosynovitis occurs concomitantly. An injection analogous to trigger finger is used (p. 44). The injection is placed at the painful area adjacent to the nodular thickening. Firm pressure may be necessary when injecting next to the fibrous tissue.

Prognosis Surgical removal of the fascial thickening is the treatment of choice. Fasciotomy and fasciectomy are usually successful in the near-term. Unfortunately, despite meticulous dissection, the condition progresses and may need reoperation with progressive contracture.

OSTEOARTHRITIS OF THE HAND

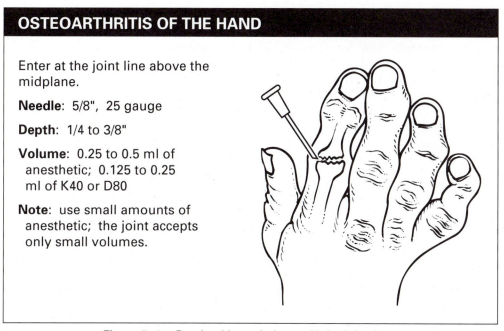

Enter at the joint line above the midplane.

Needle: 5/8", 25 gauge

Depth: 1/4 to 3/8"

Volume: 0.25 to 0.5 ml of anesthetic; 0.125 to 0.25 ml of K40 or D80

Note: use small amounts of anesthetic; the joint accepts only small volumes.

Figure 5–4. Proximal interphalangeal joint injection.

Description Osteoarthritis of the hands is a very common wear-and-tear arthritis that affects the distal interphalangeal (DIP) joints and to a lesser extent the PIP joints. It is characterized by relatively painless bony enlargement and by deformity (Heberden nodes at the DIP joints and Bouchard nodes at the PIP joints). A family history and heavy use and exposure to vibratory tools are all associated with an increased susceptibility.

Symptoms   Most patients have bony enlargement of the fingers and seek confirmation of their self-diagnosis (which is usually accurate). A minority experience finger pain and swelling in a single joint or in multiple joints.

"Am I getting what my grandma calls 'old-age arthritis'?"

"I hate my hands. They're so crooked and ugly."

"Look at my hands; I'm really getting older."

"I can't make a fist anymore; my fingers won't close."

"My hands are a little stiff in the morning, but they really don't hurt that much."

"I know I have arthritis, but my middle knuckle is so much bigger than the others and it won't bend anymore."

Exam   Each patient should be examined for bone enlargement, loss of finger flexibility, and signs of inflammation involving the DIP and PIP joints of the hand.

EXAM SUMMARY

1. Involvement of the DIP and PIP joints with bone enlargement
2. Loss of finger flexibility (inability to make a fist)
3. Relative absence of inflammatory signs (minimal evidence of synovitis)

(1) The DIP and the PIP joints of the hand have bone enlargement along the sides of the joints. The involvement is greater in the DIP joints in most cases. (2) As the disease progresses, the flexibility of the fingers gradually decreases. The patient is unable to make a fist, and extension may be lost in severe cases. The DIP joints begin to sublux to the ulnar side, all tending to create the typical deformity. (3) Inflammation and synovitis are notably absent, with the exception of a group of young women presenting with erosive osteoarthritis. This minority presents with swelling, heat, and boggy enlargement of the DIP and PIP joints. (4) The end-stage form of the disease is characterized by large, palpable bony osteophytes, decreased range of motion of the DIP and PIP joints, ankylosis of selected joints, and atrophy of the intrinsic muscles of the hand.

X-Rays   Plain films of the hand are always recommended and are diagnostic. The joint distribution can be accurately assessed. Asymmetric narrowing of the articular cartilage along with bony osteophyte formation on either side of the joint line is characteristic. Advanced cases show ever-increasing ulnar deviation, subchondral cyst formation, and ankylosis.

Diagnosis   The characteristic changes of bony enlargement with little inflammatory reaction in the typical joint distribution is highly suggestive of the diagnosis. Confirmation of the diagnosis, especially in early presentations, is made by typical changes on x-rays.

Treatment   The goals of treatment are to confirm the diagnosis, to advise on proper joint protection, and to reduce acute inflammation and swelling.

Step 1: Diagnose the condition by clinical signs and routine x-ray.

Educate the patient, "This is wear-and-tear arthritis that results from aging."

Avoid extremes of position, excessive or repetitious gripping and grasping, and vibratory tools.

Offer coated aspirin or acetaminophen as being preferable to the nonsteroidal anti-inflammatory drugs.

    Apply heat, including paraffin treatments.

    Avoid the cold.

Step 2 (weeks to years): For inflammatory flares, try simple immobilization with buddy tape (p. 176) or a tube splint (p. 176).

    A local injection of D80 or K40 can be used in selected fingers when swelling or heat is prominent.

Physical Therapy   Physical therapy plays a minor role in the overall treatment of osteoarthritis, simply because most patients do not seek medical treatment or are asymptomatic. However, application of heat to the affected joints in warm to hot water and avoidance of cold exposure are always recommended. Gentle stretch exercises in extension and toning by gentle gripping exercises (p. 149) can preserve function.

Injection Technique   Inflammatory flares in the PIP joints can be injected with good results. The DIP joints are too small to inject into (see Rheumatoid Arthritis for details, below). Note that occasionally an isolated small joint of the hand will present with enlargement and moderate-to-severe swelling (enough to interfere with flexion). The symptoms gradually develop over weeks, as opposed to an acute presentation over days seen with an acute infection. A history of trauma is often obtained. This mono-articular traumatic arthritis is an acute flare of an underlying osteoarthritic joint and is very responsive to intra-articular injection.

Prognosis   The course of osteoarthritis is extremely variable. The prognosis is determined chiefly by hereditary factors and by improper use or by overuse. Any treatment, including injection, is palliative. Surgery is rarely indicated and should be discouraged. Surgery on the small joints can lead to postoperative stiffness from peri-articular scarring. Permanent contracture can occur with surgery!

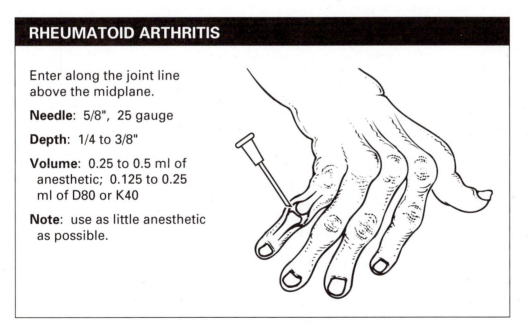

RHEUMATOID ARTHRITIS

Enter along the joint line above the midplane.

Needle: 5/8", 25 gauge

Depth: 1/4 to 3/8"

Volume: 0.25 to 0.5 ml of anesthetic; 0.125 to 0.25 ml of D80 or K40

Note: use as little anesthetic as possible.

Figure 5–5. Proximal interphalangeal joint injection.

Description   Rheumatoid arthritis (RA) is an inflammatory arthritis that can present in a variety of ways. "Classic" RA presents as a symmetric, polyarticular, small joint arthritis affecting the MCP, PIP, or MTP joints. It is characterized by fusiform swelling and by synovial thickening around these joints. "Nonclassic" RA may present in a single joint (monoarticular) or in several medium to large joints (pauciarticular) or as a fleeting, small joint arthritis that affects the small joints (palindromic). All are characterized by moderately intense inflammation and swelling.

Symptoms Depending on the presentation, the patient has joint stiffness, joint swelling, or loss of mobility of the affected joints.

"My hands have been swelling at the knuckles."

"I have to put my hands in hot running water in the morning to get rid of the horrible stiffness."

"I'm losing my grip. I can't hold on to my tools any longer."

"My hands hurt so much that it's even hard to pull up the sheets on the bed."

"My hands are so swollen that they feel like they're going to explode."

"The balls of my feet are so tender, I can't wear my shoes any longer."

"Every time I go up the stairs, the balls of my feet hurt."

"I can't bend my wrist without pain."

"My knee is swollen and feverish."

"I can't straighten my elbows all the way."

Exam Each patient should be examined for joint inflammation, swelling, and deformity along with a careful documentation of the involvement of the small, medium, and large joints of the skeleton.

EXAM SUMMARY

> 1. Early: a normal exam or subtle swelling in the MCPs, PIPs, or the MTPs
> 2. The MCP or MTP squeeze signs
> 3. Joint enlargement due to synovial thickening
> 4. Loss of joint mobility
> 5. Deformity: ulnar deviation, subluxation, hammer toes, etc.

(1) The earliest findings in RA may be so subtle or so evanescent (depending on the time of day) as to escape detection by the examiner. (2) As the condition advances, swelling appears. Squeezing the MCPs or MTPs together from side to side is a useful, quick screening sign for hand and feet involvement. (3) Otherwise, individual joints are inspected and palpated for swelling and thickening. For the small joints, this is best accomplished by alternating compression of the joint with four fingers. Two fingers are placed above and below the joint, and two fingers are placed along the sides of the joint. Pressure is applied back and forth, feeling for synovial thickening. (4) As the condition progresses, finger flexibility becomes impaired. The hand becomes doughy and loose due to ligamentous laxity. The intrinsic muscles of the hand begin to waste. (5) Ulnar deviation of the MCPs eventually develops. The hand generally loses its strength.

Early involvement of the wrist is associated with subtle swelling dorsally and obvious pain at the extremes of dorsiflexion and volarflexion. Early involvement of the elbows characteristically shows a loss of normal extension. Elbow swelling may be present laterally (the "bulge sign" appears halfway between the olecranon process and the lateral epicondyle). Early involvement of the ankle is associated with general swelling around the medial and lateral malleoli and with modest pain with plantarflexion and dorsiflexion. Knee involvement is almost always associated with effusion.

X-Rays   X-rays are always indicated. Early plain films are often normal or show only subtle juxta-articular osteoporosis. As the condition progresses, osteoporosis becomes more obvious, symmetric loss of articular cartilage develops, and joint erosions form close to the lateral margins.

Diagnosis   The diagnosis of RA may be elusive early on in the course of the disease. The diagnosis is based on the clinical findings of a symmetric, small joint pattern of stiffness, pain, and swelling (classic RA) or the demonstration of an inflammatory effusion (pauciarticular or monoarticular RA). In some cases, re-examination and re-evaluation may be necessary at 1- to 2-month intervals until the case "blossoms." Plain films of the hand can be helpful in determining the extent and severity of the disease but cannot replace the findings on exam or the clinical clues from the history. Note that the rheumatoid factor is negative in 15% of cases of RA (the so-called seronegative RA). The RA factor should *NOT* be relied on as a screening test for RA in patients presenting with arthralgia or arthritis.

Treatment   The goals of treatment are to confirm the diagnosis, to stage the extent of the disease, and to begin step care to reduce pain and inflammation.

Step 1: Confirm the diagnosis by clinical exam, x-ray, or lab work.
      Balance periods of use and limitation with stretch exercises (p. 150).
      Avoid vibrating tools, repetitive fine finger motions, and heavy gripping and grasping.
      Offer salicylates, acetaminophen or an NSAID for moderate disease.
      Heat to reduce stiffness.
      Minimize the use of narcotics.

Step 2 (months to years): Alternate between NSAIDs to maintain potency.
      Give a local injection for flares in isolated joints (rule out infection first).
      Gold salts, plaquenil, and methotrexate are given for advanced disease.
      Offer a physical and occupational therapy consultation for deformities.

Step 3 (years): Request an orthopedic consultation for joint replacement.

Physical Therapy   Physical and occupational therapy play a very important role in the overall management of RA (especially in the late stages).

PHYSICAL THERAPY SUMMARY

> 1. Heating, especially in the morning
> 2. Gentle stretch exercises to preserve range of motion
> 3. Toning exercises, especially at the large joints
> 4. Occupational therapy

Heating can be very helpful in increasing joint mobility. It is often used by the patient in the morning to reduce the morning stiffness caused by joint fluid "gelling." *Range of motion stretch exercises* are helpful to preserve function and are used extensively after joint replacement surgery. *Toning exercises* are extremely important at the large joints and are used less frequently for involvement in the small joints. For the advanced case with deformity, *occupational aides* (e.g., specialized grips, extension rods) can be extremely helpful.

Injection Technique   Local injection can be highly effective for isolated joint involvement, especially in the pauciarticular presentation of the disease or when one joint persistently swells.

Position: The hand is placed flat with the palm down and the fingers extended.

Technique: The distal metacarpal head or the distal proximal phalangeal head is
    identified. (This can be facilitated by subluxing the distal portion of the joint

dorsally.) The MCP and PIP joints are injected at the joint line above the midplane to avoid the neurovascular bundle. These small joints can only accommodate small volumes, thus anesthesia should be kept to a minimum and placed outside the joint! The 25-gauge needle is advanced down to the adjacent bone. (Note that the joint is not entered directly.) With the needle held flush against the bone, the medication is injected with moderate pressure under the synovial lining.

Restrictions: Postinjection splinting is not necessary. Modest restrictions of gripping, grasping, and pinching should be recommended for 30 days.

Prognosis   A local injection may provide weeks or even months of temporary relief, depending on the activity and progression of the disease. A progressive deformity can be treated with arthroplasty.

CHAPTER 6

Chest

COSTOCHONDRITIS

Enter on the top of the rib; angle the syringe perpendicular to the skin.

Needle: 5/8", 25 gauge

Depth: 1/2"

Volume: 1 to 2 ml of local anesthetic and 0.5 ml of either D80 or K40

Note: the injections should be placed flush against the chondral junction applying mild pressure.

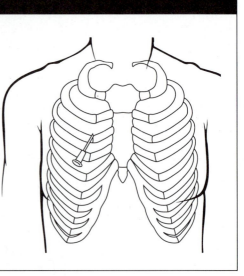

Figure 6–1. Costochondritis injection.

Description   Costochondritis is an inflammation of the cartilage of the chest wall. Irritation occurs either at the costochondral junction or at the junction of the sternum and the cartilage (costosternal syndrome). Most cases are of unproven cause (idiopathic or Tietze syndrome). A rare case follows thoracic surgery and notably open heart surgery. Almost all cases resolve spontaneously over several weeks.

Symptoms   Most patients have chest pain that is well localized to the chest wall. The pain is aggravated by external pressure. Unfortunately, patients frequently confuse this pain with coronary pain, especially those with a history of heart disease.

"I think I'm having a heart attack!"

"It hurts right here (pointing to the parasternal area with one or two fingers) whenever I cough or take a deep breath."

"I can't sleep on my left side at night. . . . Whenever I roll over onto my side, I get this sharp pain in my chest."

"Ever since my bypass, I've had this sharp pain along the side of my incision."

"Coughing just kills me."

"It's like there is sandpaper between the ends of my ribs. It feels like the flesh has pulled away from the bone."

Exam   Each patient should be examined for localized irritation at the costochondral or the sternochondral junctions.

EXAM SUMMARY

1. Localized tenderness either 1" from the midline of the sternum or at the costochondral junction
2. A positive result on a rib compression test
3. Regional anesthetic block just over the cartilage

(1) Localized tenderness is present either at the junction of the sternum and the

costal cartilage or at the junction between the rib and the costal cartilage. The intercostal spaces should be nontender. The sternochondral junctions are ¾ to 1″ lateral to the midline. The costochondral junctions vary from 3 to 4″ from the midline. (2) The rib compression test result is positive. Pressure either from the anteroposterior direction or from either side reproduces the discomfort. (3) The diagnosis is confirmed by a regional anesthetic block just at the top of the cartilage.

X-Rays   Routine chest x-rays and plain films of the ribs are not necessary for the diagnosis; however, the patient's expectations for special testing are always high. A chest x-ray, rib films, and even a T spine series are often ordered. No specific changes are seen on these tests.

Diagnosis   The diagnosis is suggested by a history of localized chest pain and by an exam showing local tenderness aggravated by chest compression. The diagnosis is confirmed by a regional anesthetic block. The latter is particularly useful in the patient with heart disease who is having difficulties accepting the diagnosis of a noncoronary problem.

Treatment   The goals of treatment are to reassure the patient that this is not a life-threatening heart problem and to reduce the local inflammation.

Step 1: Educate the patient, "This is not a heart pain" and "Most cases resolve on their own!"
>   Observe for 2 to 3 weeks.
>   A cough suppressant is given when indicated.
>   A rib binder or a neoprene waist wrap (p. 178) or a snug-fitting bra (do not use for the debilitated or for patients older than 65 years of age).
>   Restrict lying on the sides, lifting, and strenuous activity.

Step 2 (3 to 4 weeks): Give a local anesthetic block plus ½ ml of K40 or D80.
>   Continue the restrictions.

Step 3 (6 to 8 weeks): Repeat the injection in 6 weeks.
>   Combine the injection with a rib binder.
>   Continue the restrictions.

Physical Therapy   Physical therapy does not have a significant role in the treatment of costochondritis. Phonophoresis with a hydrocortisone gel has questionable value.

Injection Technique   A local injection of the chondral junctions can assist in confirming the diagnosis and may dramatically alter the course of the condition.

Position: The patient is placed in the supine position.

Technique: The point of maximum tenderness at the top of the cartilage is palpated.
>   The center point of the cartilage is identified by placing one finger above and one finger below the cartilage in the intercostal spaces. The skin is entered and anesthetized. The syringe is held perpendicular to the skin and advanced ½ to ¾″ down to the firm resistance of the cartilage. One to 2 ml of anesthetic followed by ½ ml of K40 or D80 is injected flush against the cartilage.

Restrictions: Lying on the sides is absolutely restricted for the next 3 days.
>   Lifting and strenuous activities are restricted for the next 30 days.
>   Use of a rib binder for 3 to 7 days can be combined with the repeat corticosteroid injection.

Prognosis   Most cases resolve spontaneously without residual. A few patients experience prolonged symptoms. A local corticosteroid injection can provide excellent palliation of symptoms.

CHAPTER 7

Back

LUMBOSACRAL STRAIN

The point of maximum muscle tenderness is identified, and the needle enters perpendicular to the skin.

Needle: 1 1/2", 22 gauge

Depth: 1 to 1 1/2"

Volume: 4 to 5 ml of anesthetic; 1 ml of D80 or K40

Note: lightly advance the needle to feel the outer fascia of the muscle; then enter the body of the muscle.

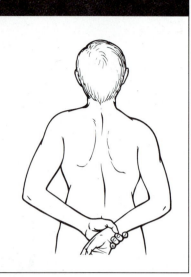

Figure 7–1. Acute low back strain.

Description Lumbosacral (LS) strain is a spasm and irritation of the supporting muscles of the lumbar spine. Overuse of improperly stretched and toned muscles, scoliosis, spondylolisthesis, osteoarthritis, previous compression fracture, or radiculopathy are underlying causes.

Symptoms The patient complains of back pain and stiffness that are well localized to the lower lumbar area.

"Oh, my aching back."

"My back is so stiff in the morning I can hardly straighten up. . . . It takes a long, hot shower to loosen up."

"I used to be able to bend over and touch my toes."

"I get these terrible back spasms right here (using the hand to rub the side of the lower back)."

"I can't sit for very long before my back starts aching."

"I can't find a comfortable chair to sit in anymore. . . . I've tried everything from hard backs to recliners."

"I can't bend forward without my back killing me."

"I can't find a comfortable position in bed, let alone a comfortable mattress."

Exam Each patient should be examined for the degree of paraspinal muscle spasm and irritation along with an assessment of loss of range of motion of the back.

EXAM SUMMARY

1. Paraspinal muscle tenderness and spasm
2. "Straightened" LS curve
3. Loss of LS flexion and lateral bending
4. A normal neurologic exam, unless there is concomitant radiculopathy

(1) The maximum paraspinal muscle tightening is 1½″ off the midline, adjacent to L3-L4. A second common trigger point is at the origin of the erector spinae, just above the sacroiliac joint. (2) The normal LS lordotic curve is "straightened" with severe muscle spasm. If the strain is unilateral, the back may tilt to the affected side (an "acquired" and reversible scoliosis). (3) Measurements of LS flexion and lateral bending are impaired. The Schober test, measuring LS flexion, is abnormal. With the patient standing as erect as possible, 10 cm is marked in the midline just above a line drawn between the iliac crests. The patient is asked to flex forward at the waist. Symptoms are noted as the patient bends forward. At full LS flexion, the marks are remeasured. A 50% increase to 15 cm is normal. Measurements of lateral bending may be abnormal as well. Normally, 20 cm measured above the iliac crests should increase to 26 cm (a 33% increase) and should be comparable with the contralateral side. (4) The neurologic exam of the lower extremity should be normal, unless concomitant radiculopathy is present.

X-Rays   An LS spine series is always recommended. Plain films of an uncomplicated lumbar strain are normal; however, many cases are accompanied by an underlying structural process, such as an old compression fracture, scoliosis, spondylolisthesis. Special testing with computed tomography (CT) scanning or magnetic resonance imaging (MRI) scanning is indicated when the local LS symptoms are associated with radicular symptoms down the leg (see Lumbar Radiculopathy, p. 63).

Diagnosis   The diagnosis is based on the localized pain, tenderness, and spasm in the lower back as long as an acute underlying processes (e.g., acute compression fracture, radiculopathy, epidural processes) are excluded. If there are any atypical features to simple lumbar strain, a work-up for an underlying process should be initiated.

Treatment   The goals of therapy are to reduce the acute erector spinae muscle spasm, to avoid aggravation of muscle spasm by stretching and toning exercises, and to treat any underlying structural back condition.

Step 1: Thoroughly examine the back and perform a complete lower extremity neurologic exam; perform plain x-rays, and order a CT scan or an MRI scan if any radicular symptoms are present (p. 63).

Avoid twisting and extremes of bending and tilting.

Advise on proper lifting with the knees: hold the object close to the body; bend at the knee and not with the back; never lift in a twisted position.

Carry heavier objects close to the body.

Reinforce an erect posture; suggest a lumbar support for the office chair and vehicle.

Begin gentle stretch exercises to maintain flexibility (p. 153).

Take a muscle relaxant at night.

The nonsteroidal anti-inflammatory drugs have limited benefit, because inflammation is not a significant part of the process.

Conserve use of narcotics for the first week.

Apply ice, alternating with heat.

Do an ultrasound for deep heating.

Use crutches if pain and spasm are severe.

Take 3 to 4 days of bedrest for the acute, severe case.

Step 2 (2 to 4 weeks): Re-evaluate the neurologic exam and back motion.

Begin strengthening exercises (p. 156).

Begin aerobics, low-impact walking, or swimming.

Reduce the use of medication.

Step 3 (6 to 8 weeks): Either resume normal activities gradually, but with continued attention to proper care of the back,

or use an LS corset for external support (pp. 178 to 179),

or, for chronic symptoms, order a transcutaneous electrical nerve stimulator (TENS) unit; consider use of a tricyclic antidepressant; or refer to a pain clinic.

Physical Therapy   Physical therapy is a fundamental part of the treatment of acute low back strain and is the main treatment for rehabilitation and prevention.

PHYSICAL THERAPY SUMMARY

> **1.** Ice or heat
> **2.** Aerobic exercises
> **3.** Stretching exercises for erector spinae, the SI joint, and the glutei
> **4.** Toning exercise
> **5.** Traction

ACUTELY   Cold, heat, and gentle stretch exercises are used in the early treatment of lumbar strain to reduce acute muscular spasm and increase lumbar flexibility.

Cold, heat, or cold alternating with heat are effective in reducing pain and muscular spasm. Recommendations are based on individual clinical responses. *Stretching exercises* are fundamental for maintaining flexibility, especially in patients with structural back disease. Side bends, knee-chest pulls, and pelvic rocks are designed to stretch the paraspinal muscles, the gluteus muscles, and the sacroiliac joints (p. 153). These exercises should be started after the hyperacute symptoms have resolved. Stretching is performed after heating the body. Initially, these exercises should be performed while the patient is lying down. As pain and muscular spasm ease, stretching can be performed while the patient is standing. Sets of 20 of each exercise are performed to the point at which the patient experiences mild discomfort.

RECOVERY/REHABILITATION   To continue the recovery process and to reduce the possibility of a recurrence, toning exercises are added at 3 to 4 weeks. *Toning exercises* are performed after the acute muscular spasms have subsided. Modified sit-ups, weighted side bends, and gentle extension exercises (p. 156) are performed after heating and stretching. Aerobic exercise is one of the best ways to prevent recurrent back strain. Walking, light jogging, swimming, or cross-country ski machine work-outs are excellent fitness exercises that will be less likely to aggravate the back.

Traction is used infrequently for acute LS strain. Patients with acute facet syndrome or persistent acute lumbar strain (despite home bedrest, medication, physical therapy) may respond dramatically to 25 to 35 lb of lumbar traction in bed. In addition, traction can be used at home in combination with traditional stretching exercises (p. 153). *Vertical traction* can be achieved by leaning against a countertop, suspending between two bar stools, or with inversion equipment. The weight of the body is used to pull the lumbar segments apart. It is used primarily for prevention. It is not appropriate for hyperacute strain. Chronic cases unresponsive to traditional stretching and toning may require a *TENS* unit for control of chronic pain.

Injection Technique   A local injection of the paraspinal muscles or the lumbar facet joints has questionable value. Occasionally, a patient will present with very localized tenderness in the erector spinae and will respond dramatically to local anesthesia or to corticosteroid injection. Note that a local injection of the paraspinal muscles should be considered only after a treatable structural process has been treated or reasonably excluded!

Position: The patient is placed completely flat in the prone position.

Technique: The point of maximum muscle tenderness is palpated. A 22-gauge 1½″ needle is passed vertically down to the outer fascia of the muscle, approximately 1 to 1¼″ deep. The muscle is entered three times in an area that is the size of a quarter. A total of 4 or 5 ml of local anesthetic is injected. The needle is withdrawn, and the local tenderness is re-evaluated. A local anesthetic injection is sufficient in most cases. It can be combined with D80 in selected cases.

Restrictions: Postinjection restriction must be tailored to the patient's condition. Three days of bed rest may be advised for acute, severe spasms. Moderate rest is recommended for patients with less severe symptoms. Prolonged walking or standing, lifting, and twisting should be restricted until clear-cut improvement is noted.

Prognosis The course of low back strain is dependent on the underlying cause and on the patient's willingness to do regular exercises. Patients with persistent symptoms require evaluation for an underlying spinous process (often an L4-L5 disk or spinal stenosis). Surgery is indicated only for these underlying conditions.

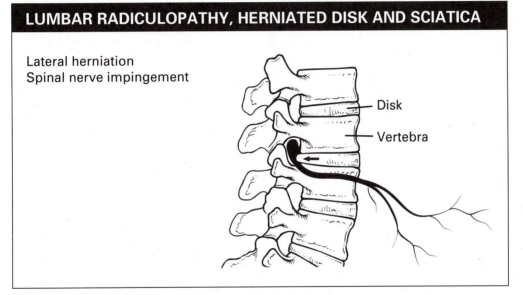

LUMBAR RADICULOPATHY, HERNIATED DISK AND SCIATICA

Lateral herniation
Spinal nerve impingement

Disk

Vertebra

Figure 7–2. Herniated disk of the lumbar spine.

Description Sciatica is the common term used to describe the pain associated with the abnormal function of the LS nerve roots or of one of the nerves of the LS plexus. Pressure on the nerve from a herniated disk, from bony osteophytes (spinal stenosis), a compression fracture, or any other extrinsic pressure (e.g., epidural process, pelvic mass, ''wallet sciatica'') causes progressive sensory, sensorimotor, or sensorimotor visceral loss.

Symptoms The patient has pain around the buttock area or pain traveling a variable distance down the lateral or posterior leg. Depending on the degree of nerve compression, the patient may also describe a loss or an abnormal sensation in the feet, weakness or clumsiness of the lower leg, or in extreme cases loss of control of bowel or bladder function.

''I have this shooting pain down my leg. It starts in my hip and goes all the way to my toes.''

''My feet feel like they're coming out of Novocain, they're tingling.''

''I'm dragging my leg.''

''My leg seems weak.''

"If I cough, I get this electric-like shock down my leg."

"If I sit too long, my toes go numb."

"It feels as if I have this burning steel rod in the center of my calf."

Exam   Each patient should be examined for the degree of lower extremity neurologic impairment, along with an evaluation of its underlying cause.

EXAM SUMMARY

---

1. Abnormal straight leg raise
2. Percussion tenderness over the spinous processes
3. Abnormal neurologic exam: sensory loss, loss of deep tendon reflex, motor weakness, loss of bowel or bladder control
4. Signs of LS strain
5. Signs reflecting the underlying cause

---

(1) The hallmark of sciatica is an abnormal straight leg-raising sign. The maneuver should be reproducible in a given position and angle and should reproduce the patient's radicular symptoms in the lower extremity. Forced dorsiflexion of the ankle may be necessary to bring out subtle signs. (2) Percussion tenderness over the spinous processes may be present in acute herniated disks, epidural processes, and other acute vertebral bony processes; however, it is an unreliable sign in spinal stenosis or any process that is outside the vertebral column. (3) Neurologically, loss of sensation in a radicular pattern is the most subtle and earliest sign of nerve dysfunction. Light touch, pinprick, and two-point discrimination are lost early. Advanced conditions may also show loss of deep tendon reflexes, loss of strength of involved muscle groups (foot dorsiflexion and plantarflexion most commonly), or loss of bowel and urinary control (cauda equina syndrome). (4) Signs of LS muscular strain may accompany sciatica (p. 60). Local paraspinous muscle tenderness and spasm and loss of normal LS flexibility may be present. (5) Finally, signs reflecting the underlying process must be sought if the primary process is not readily evident at the spinal level.

X-Rays   An LS spine series is always recommended; however, plain films of the spine are not very effective in determining the cause of sciatica. Spinal stenosis requires CT scanning. Epidural processes and herniated disks require the fine anatomic detail of MRI scanning. Elusive cases may need an electromyogram (EMG) to evaluate for nerve root dysfunction.

Diagnosis   The diagnosis of sciatica is often based solely on the description of a radicular pain described by the patient. One of the best neurologic correlates is the patient's own description of the location of the radicular pattern: down the posterior leg (L5-S1) or down the lateral leg (L4-L5). The neurologic examination is used to stage the severity of the problem (e.g., sensory, motor, visceral). However, the definitive diagnosis requires specialized testing!

Treatment   The goals of treatment are to confirm the diagnosis, to reduce the pressure over the nerve, to improve neurologic function, to reduce any accompanying low back strain, and to evaluate for the need for surgery.

Step 1: Thoroughly examine the back and the lower extremity neurologic function.

Perform x-rays or order a CT scan or an MRI scan.

Order bedrest for 3 to 5 days for acute symptoms.

Limit walking and standing for 30 to 45 minutes each day.

Advocate use of crutches so that the patient can get from bed to the bathroom.

Use a strong muscle relaxer and an appropriate dose of a potent narcotic.
Apply ice.

Hospitalize and consult with a neurosurgeon if the patient has bilateral symptoms, extreme motor weakness, or incontinence of stool or urine.

Step 2 (7 to 14 days): Re-evaluate the patient's neurologic and back exam.

Begin gentle stretch exercises while the patient is in bed (p. 153).

Use hand-held weights in bed to keep the upper body toned.

Liberalize the amount of time spent out of bed, still relying on crutches.

Use a simple LS corset while out of bed (p. 178).

Step 3 (2 to 3 weeks): Re-evaluate the patient.

Reduce the use of medications.

Begin toning exercises of the lower back (p. 156).

Advise swimming to tone muscles and recondition the cardiovascular system.

Emphasize proper care of the back (p. 155).

Step 4 (3 to 6 weeks): Order a neurosurgical consultation if symptoms persist or progress.

Nonsurgical candidates may need an LS elastic binder (p. 179).

Physical Therapy   Physical therapy is a integral part of active treatment and prevention of recurrent sciatica (see Low Back Strain, p. 62). Greater emphasis is placed on bedrest for the hyperacute symptoms, on crutches to assist in ambulation, and on general muscular toning when at bedrest.

Injection Technique   An epidural injection of anesthetic and corticosteroid can be given in persistent cases of sciatica (sensory symptoms only!). This procedure should be performed by an anesthesiologist or an interventional radiologist.

Prognosis   Patients with sensory complaints only or very minimal motor findings do very well with medical treatment. The vast majority (75 to 80%) respond to nonsurgical conservative therapy. Surgical consultation is always indicated for progressive neurologic deficits, large disk herniations associated with dramatic motor loss or incontinence, fragmented disks with fragments lodged in the neuroforamina, and in patients with persistent sensorimotor symptoms that correspond with the anatomic abnormalities on scan. Diskectomy, laminectomy, decompression, and fusion are the various procedures that can be performed.

CHAPTER 8

Hip

TROCHANTERIC BURSITIS

Enter over the midtrochanter in the lateral decubitus position; advance perpendicular to the skin down to the gluteus medius tendon; then continue to the bone.

Needle: 1 1/2", 22 gauge or a 22-gauge spinal needle

Depth: 1 1/4" to 2 1/2"

Volume: 4 ml of anesthetic; 1 ml of K40

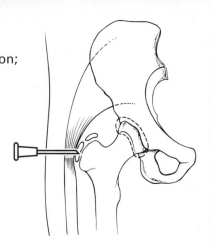

Figure 8–1. Trochanteric bursa injection.

Description   Trochanteric bursitis is an inflammation of the lubricating sac located between the midportion of the trochanteric process of the femur and the gluteus medius tendon/iliotibial tract. Repetitive or uneven contracture of the gluteus medius and direct pressure over the trochanteric process are the two most common aggravating factors. An underlying back, sacroiliac, or lower leg gait disturbance are predisposing conditions.

Symptoms   The patient complains of hip pain over the outer thigh or difficulty with walking.

"Whenever I roll over onto my right side, this sharp pain in my hip wakes me up."

"I get this achy pain in my hip (pointing to the upper outer thigh) when I walk too much in the mall."

"I can't stand very long."

"I have this sharp pain in my hip (pointing to the outer thigh) that I feel clear down (the outside of my leg) to my knee."

"Climbing up the stairs has become impossible."

"My back has hurt me for years. Lately, I've had a sharper pain right here (pointing to the upper outer thigh) whenever I lie on a hard surface."

Exam   Each patient should be examined for the degree of local irritation at the greater trochanter along with an assessment of gait, the lower back, and the sacroiliac joints.

EXAM SUMMARY

1. Local midtrochanteric tenderness
2. Aggravation of pain at the extremes of hip rotation (mild)
3. Pain aggravated by isometric hip abduction (25% of cases)
4. Normal range of motion of the hip
5. Associated gait disturbance, leg-length discrepancy, back or sacroiliac condition

(1) Local tenderness is present at the midportion of the greater trochanter. This is best identified in the lateral decubitus position. The maximum tenderness is 1½″ below the superior portion of the trochanter, directly over the maximum lateral prominence. (2) Stiffness or mild discomfort may be experienced at the extremes of internal or external rotation of the hip. This is present in approximately 50% of cases. (3) Isometrically resisted hip abduction may aggravate the pain in 25% of cases. (4) The range of motion of the hip in an uncomplicated case should be normal. (5) Signs of an underlying leg-length discrepancy, gait disturbance, or an underlying back or sacroiliac condition should be examined for.

X-Rays   X-rays of the hip are strongly recommended. Plain films of the pelvis and hip may show calcification (in a few patients) but are used mainly to exclude underlying degenerative arthritis, pelvic tilting due to a short leg, or the rare case of a bony lesion. Bone scanning, computed tomography (CT) scanning, or magnetic resonance imaging (MRI) scanning are also used to exclude underlying conditions at the lumbosacral spine, sacroiliac joint, or the femur.

Diagnosis   The diagnosis of an uncomplicated case of trochanteric bursitis is based on the clinical findings of outer thigh pain, local tenderness at the midtrochanter, and pain relief with regional anesthetic block. Regional anesthetic block may be very helpful in differentiating the pain of trochanteric bursitis from the referred pain from the gluteus medius bursa (p. 71), the lumbosacral spine, or the dysesthetic pain of meralgia paresthetica (p. 76). Complicated cases with a suspected underlying cause require specialized testing for a definitive diagnosis.

Treatment   The goals of treatment are to reduce the inflammation in the bursa, to correct any underlying disturbance of gait, and to prevent a recurrence by proper hip and back stretch exercises.

Step 1: Evaluate and correct any underlying gait disturbance (e.g., shoe lift, low back stretch exercises, a knee brace, custom-made foot orthotics).

Reduce weightbearing (e.g., a lean bar, sitting versus standing, crutches temporarily, weight loss).

Restrict repetitious bending (e.g., climbing stairs, getting out of a chair).

Avoid direct pressure.

Do daily stretch exercises for the gluteus medius (p. 158).

Take a nonsteroidal anti-inflammatory drug (e.g., ibuprofen [Advil, Motrin]) for 4 weeks.

Step 2 (6 to 8 weeks): For persistent symptoms, re-evaluate for an underlying cause (e.g., CT scan of the back, bone scan).

X-ray the hip and pelvis (standing anteroposterior pelvis, for leg length discrepancy).

Inject the bursa with K40.

Repeat the injection in 4 to 6 weeks if symptoms have not decreased by 50%.

Step 3 (10 to 12 weeks): With improvement, emphasize stretch exercises for the hip and back.

Avoid direct pressure.

Use deep ultrasound for persistent cases.

Recommend a transcutaneous electrical nerve stimulation (TENS) unit for persistent cases.

Physical Therapy   Physical therapy plays an important role in the active treatment of trochanteric bursitis and a major role in preventing a recurrence.

ACUTELY/RECOVERY   Heat treatments and passive stretch exercises are used in the first few weeks to reduce the pressure over the bursal sac.

PHYSICAL THERAPY SUMMARY

> **1.** Heat
> **2.** Stretch exercises for the gluteus medius
> **3.** Stretch exercises for the low back and sacroiliac joints
> **4.** Ultrasound
> **5.** TENS unit

Heat is applied to the outer thigh for 15 to 20 minutes to prepare the area for stretching. *Stretch exercises of the gluteus medius tendon* are recommended to reduce the pressure over the bursa. While in the sitting position, cross-leg pulls are performed in sets of 20 (p. 158). The maximum amount of stretch is obtained when the buttock is kept flat. These are followed by *low back and sacroiliac stretches* (p. 153). Stretching all three areas provides flexibility through the lower spine, the sacroiliac joints, and the hips. *Ultrasound* deep heating can be combined with stretching. A TENS unit may be necessary for patients with chronic bursitis secondary to structural back disease or chronic neurologic impairment.

REHABILITATION   Several weeks after the local symptoms have resolved, daily stretch exercises are reduced to three times a week. Maintaining low back, sacroiliac, and hip flexibility will lessen the chance of recurrent bursitis.

Injection Technique   For an uncomplicated bursitis (i.e., not associated with a correctable underlying cause), local injection is the treatment of choice.

Position: The patient is placed in the lateral decubitus position with the affected side up and the knees flexed to 90 degrees.

Technique: The midtrochanter is identified. The needle is centered over the mid-trochanter and advanced vertically to the firm resistance of the gluteus medius tendon. One milliliter of anesthetic is placed at the tendon and then passed down to the bone (the patient will experience sharp pain as soon as the needle touches the periosteum!). The medication is injected with the needle held close to the bone, 1 to 2 mm above (firm pressure may be needed). The patient is re-examined. If the local tenderness over the trochanter is significantly relieved, then 1 ml of K40 is injected. The bursa is massaged for 5 minutes after the injection is given.

Restrictions: The patient is advised to restrict activities for 3 days and to avoid prolonged standing and walking for the next 30 days.

Prognosis   Uncomplicated cases of bursitis usually respond dramatically to one or two injections 6 weeks apart. A poor response to an injection suggests either a chronic bursal thickening or an undiscovered underlying cause. The prognosis for recovery depends greatly on the underlying cause, the patient's willingness to do stretch exercises, and the degree of obesity. Intractable symptoms are seen in severe obesity, severe structural back disease, and patients with chronic neurologic impairment. Bursectomy is rarely advised.

GLUTEUS MEDIUS BURSITIS

Enter 1" above the superior aspect of the greater trochanter in the lateral decubitus position; advance down to the gluteus medius tendon; then to the tip of the bone.

Needle: 1 1/2", 22 gauge or a 22-gauge spinal needle

Depth: 1 1/4" to 2 1/2"

Volume: 4 ml of anesthetic; 1 ml of K40

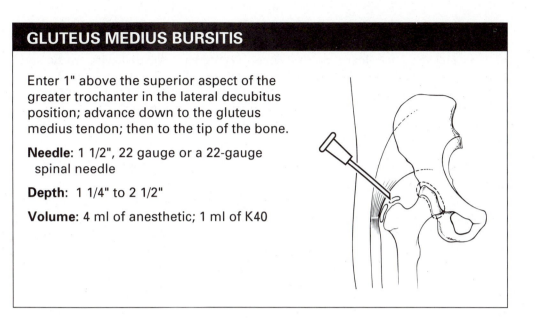

Figure 8–2.   Gluteus medius bursitis injection.

Description   Gluteus medius bursitis (also referred to as the deep trochanteric bursitis) is an inflammation of the bursal sac that is located between the top of the superior trochanteric process and the gluteus medius tendon. It serves to lubricate the gluteus medius tendon, the piriformis insertion, and the bone. Repetitive flexing of the hip and direct pressure aggravate this condition.

Symptoms   The patient complains of hip pain or difficulties with walking (identical to Trochanteric Bursitis, p. 68).

"Whenever I roll over onto my right side, this sharp pain in my hip wakes me up."

"I get this achy pain in my hip (pointing to the upper outer thigh) when I walk too much in the mall."

"I can't stand very long."

"I have this sharp pain in my hip (pointing to the outer thigh) that I feel right down (the outside of my leg) to my knee."

"Climbing up the stairs has become impossible."

"My back has hurt me for years. Lately, I've had a sharper pain right here (pointing to the upper outer thigh) whenever I lie on a hard surface."

Exam   Each patient should be examined for the degree of local irritation at the top of the greater trochanter and the range of motion of the hip, along with an assessment of gait, the lower back, and the sacroiliac joints.

EXAM SUMMARY

1. Local tenderness above the trochanteric process
2. Pain aggravated at the extremes of hip rotation
3. Pain aggravated by isometric hip abduction (75% of cases)
4. Normal range of motion of the hip
5. Associated gait disturbance, leg-length discrepancy, or back or sacroiliac condition

(1) Maximum tenderness is located just superior to the trochanteric process of the femur in the midline. This is best identified with the patient in the lateral decubitus position and the knee flexed to 90 degrees. (2) When compared with trochanteric bursitis, pain is more often aggravated by the extremes of hip rotation and (3) when resisting hip abduction isometrically. (4) The range of motion of the hip is normal in an uncomplicated case. (5) Frequently, there is an associated gait disturbance, leg-length discrepancy, or back or sacroiliac condition.

X-Rays   X-rays of the hip and pelvis are recommended. Plain films of the pelvis and hip may show calcification (in a few cases) arthritis of the hip, or abnormalities of the sacroiliac joints or the lumbosacral spine. Uncomplicated cases do not require any specialized testing. However, when an underlying cause is suggested on clinical grounds, bone scanning, CT scanning, or MRI scanning may be necessary to evaluate the integrity of the femur or to obtain greater detail at the sacroiliac joints or the lumbar spine.

Diagnosis   The diagnosis is based on the clinical findings of lateral thigh pain, local tenderness at the superior trochanteric process, and pain relief with regional anesthetic block. Regional anesthetic block at the superior trochanteric process will differentiate trochanteric bursitis from gluteus medius bursitis, the pain of lumbosacral radiculopathy, and the referred pain from the sacroiliac joint. Again, complicated cases may require special testing to exclude an underlying cause.

Treatment   The goals of treatment are to reduce the inflammation in the bursal sac, to correct any underlying disturbance of gait, and to prevent a recurrence by proper hip and back stretch exercises.

Step 1: Evaluate and correct any underlying gait disturbance (e.g., shoe lift, low back stretching exercises, a knee brace, custom-made foot orthotics).

Reduce weightbearing (e.g., a lean bar, sitting versus standing, crutches temporarily, weight loss).

Restrict repetitious bending (e.g., climbing stairs, getting out of a chair).

Avoid direct pressure.

Do daily stretch exercises for the gluteus medius (p. 158).

Suggest a nonsteroidal anti-inflammatory drug (e.g., ibuprofen [Advil, Motrin]) for 4 weeks.

Step 2 (6 to 8 weeks): For persistent symptoms, re-evaluate for an underlying cause (e.g., a CT scan of the back, bone scan of the femur).

X-ray the hip and pelvis (standing anteroposterior pelvis for leg-length discrepancy).

Inject the bursa with K40.

Repeat the injection in 4 to 6 weeks if symptoms have not been reduced by 50%.

Suggest 7 to 14 days of touch-down weightbearing with crutches for difficult cases and for those associated with gait disturbance.

Step 3 (10 to 12 weeks): With improvement, emphasize stretch exercises for the hip and back.

Avoid direct pressure.

Apply deep ultrasound for persistent cases.

Use a TENS unit for persistent cases.

Physical Therapy   Physical therapy plays an important role in the active treatment of gluteus medius bursitis and a major role in preventing recurrence.

PHYSICAL THERAPY SUMMARY

> **1.** Heat
> **2.** Stretch exercises for the gluteus medius
> **3.** Stretch exercises for the low back and sacroiliac joints
> **4.** Ultrasound
> **5.** A TENS unit

ACUTELY/RECOVERY Heat treatments and passive stretch exercises are used in the first few weeks to reduce the pressure over the bursal sac. *Heat* is applied to the outer thigh for 15 to 20 minutes to prepare the area for stretching. *Stretch exercises of the gluteus medius* are recommended to reduce the pressure over the bursa. While in the sitting position, cross-leg pulls are performed in sets of 20 (p. 158). The maximum amount of stretch is obtained when the buttock is kept flat. These exercises are followed by *low back and sacroiliac stretches* (p. 153). Stretching all three areas provides flexibility through the lower spine, the sacroiliac joints, and the hips. *Ultrasound* deep heating can be combined with stretching. A *TENS* unit may be necessary for cases of chronic bursitis secondary to structural back disease or chronic neurologic impairment.

REHABILITATION Several weeks after the local symptoms have resolved, daily stretch exercises are reduced to three times a week. Maintaining low back and sacroiliac and hip flexibility will reduce the chance of recurrent bursitis.

Injection Technique For an uncomplicated bursitis (i.e., not associated with a correctable underlying cause), local injection is the treatment of choice.

Position: The patient is placed in the lateral decubitus position with the affected side up. The knees are flexed to 90 degrees.

Technique: The superior trochanter is identified, and the midline of the femur is estimated. The needle enters 1″ above the center of the superior trochanter and is advanced at a 45-degree angle down to the firm resistance of the gluteus medius tendon. One milliliter of anesthetic is placed at the tendon, and then the needle is passed another ½″ down to the periosteum of the femur (the patient will experience sharp pain as soon as the needle touches the periosteum!). Note that if bone is not encountered within ¾″, the needle should be withdrawn through the gluteus medius tendon and redirected either more superficially in an asthenic patient or deeper in a well-padded patient! Medication is injected with the needle held close to the femur, 1 to 2 mm above (firm pressure may be needed when injecting). If the local tenderness over the trochanter is significantly relieved, then 1 ml of K40 is injected. The bursa is massaged for 5 minutes after the injection.

Restrictions: Activities should be restricted for 3 days, and prolonged standing and walking should be avoided for the next 30 days. Crutches can be used for 7 to 14 days for persistent cases and for those associated with a fixed gait disturbance.

Prognosis Uncomplicated cases of bursitis usually respond dramatically to one or two injections 6 weeks apart. A poor response to an injection suggests either a chronic bursal thickening or an undiscovered underlying cause. The prognosis for recovery depends greatly on the underlying cause, the patient's willingness to do stretch exercises, and the degree of obesity. Intractable symptoms are seen in severe obesity, severe structural back disease, and patients with chronic neurologic impairment especially associated with a fixed gait disturbance (e.g., polio, Parkinson disease, previous stroke). Bursectomy is not advised.

OSTEOARTHRITIS OF THE HIP

A hip prosthesis is in place.

Indication: intractable pain; loss of function; older than 62 years of age; loss of internal rotation; protrusio acetabulae

A hip joint injection is rarely indicated.

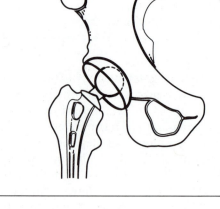

Figure 8–3. Hip prosthesis.

Description   Osteoarthritis of the hip is a wear-and-tear of the articular cartilage of the head of the femur and the acetabulum. Obesity, a family history, a history of systemic arthritis, and a history of a severe gait disturbance are predisposing factors.

Symptoms   The patient has groin or thigh pain or loss of mobility.

"I can't get my socks on anymore . . . and there's absolutely no way I can tie my shoe laces."

"My hip is getting stiffer and stiffer."

"My right hip is beginning to hurt just like the left hip did before I had it replaced."

"I can't walk through the mall any longer without having to stop two or three times (because of hip pain)."

"I've had this deep achy pain (pointing to the anterior hip) whenever I walk a certain distance."

"I can't believe that I have arthritis in my hip. My hip has never hurt me. I feel pain in my lower thigh and knee. I thought I had arthritis in my knee."

Exam   Each patient should have the general function of the hip and lower extremities examined, along with specific measurements of the range of motion of the hip.

EXAM SUMMARY

1. Functional loss of normal gait; unable to remove socks; can't cross legs
2. Loss of internal and external rotation with end-point stiffness
3. A positive Fabere maneuver
4. Tenderness 1 to ½" below the inguinal ligament

(1) General hip function can be assessed by observing gait, the transfer from a chair to the exam table, the removal of the shoes and socks, or crossing the legs. As arthritis advances, these basic functions become more and more difficult to accomplish. (2) The range of motion of the hip is restricted. Early disease shows a loss of internal rotation and end-point stiffness. As the condition progresses, external rotation is lost as well. Normally, a 50-year-old patient should have 45 degrees of internal and external rotation. (3) The result of the Fabere maneuver (also known as Patrick test) may be positive. The hip is placed in *flexion*, *ab*duction, and *ex*ternal rotation (a figure-of-four position), and pressure is applied to the anterior superior iliac spine and the knee. This stretches the anterior capsule of the hip and causes pain. (4) Tenderness may be found 1 to ½″ below the midportion of the inguinal ligament (very close to the femoral artery). Note that all of these findings on exam are exaggerated with inflammatory arthritis, severe with avascular necrosis of the hip, and extreme with acute septic arthritis.

X-Rays   X-rays of the hip are always indicated. Plain films of the hip show loss of joint space between the superior acetabulum and the femoral head (normally 6 to 8 mm), increased bony sclerosis of the superior acetabulum, osteophyte formation along the superior acetabulum, and subchondral cyst formation in advanced cases. A standing anteroposterior pelvis is an excellent study to assess for arthritic change at either hip, protrusio acetabulae, and pelvic tilting due to a short lower extremity or to loss of joint space.

Diagnosis   The diagnosis is based on the loss of hip rotation coupled with characteristic changes on plain films of the hip.

Treatment   The goals of treatment are to relieve pain, preserve function, and stage for surgery.

Step 1: Measure the patient's loss of internal and external rotation (normally 40 to 45 degrees in a 50 year old), obtain plain x-rays, and determine their baseline functional status.

Advise on passive hip stretch exercises (p. 157) to preserve range of motion.

Prescribe a nonsteroidal anti-inflammatory drug (e.g., ibuprofen [Advil, Motrin]) in full dose. Emphasize the need to take it regularly for its anti-inflammatory effect.

Restrict jogging, Jazzercise, and other impact exercises.

Suggest padded insoles to reduce impact pressure (p. 185).

Step 2 (months to years): Remeasure hip rotation and evaluate functional status.

X-ray again if rotation has decreased by more than 20% or if function has changed dramatically.

Consider switching to another nonsteroidal anti-inflammatory drug.

Use narcotics cautiously!

Step 3 (months to years): Orthopedic consultation when (1) pain is intractable, (2) function is severely limited, (3) internal rotation has declined to 10 to 15 degrees, or (4) protrusio acetabulae has developed. Assess the patient's surgical candidacy!

Physical Therapy   Physical therapy plays an adjunctive role in the overall treatment of osteoarthritis of the hip.

PHYSICAL THERAPY SUMMARY

1. Stretch exercises of the adductors, rotators, and glutei
2. Toning exercises of iliopsoas and the glutei
3. Occupational therapy consultation

ACUTELY/RECOVERY Stretching and toning exercises are recommended to maintain hip flexibility and to preserve the muscular tone. Figure-of-four, Indian-style sitting, and knee-chest pulls are performed daily in sets of 20 to stretch the adductors, rotators, and gluteus muscles (p. 157). Toning exercises of the iliopsoas and the gluteus follow the stretch exercises. Initially, straight leg raises are performed without weights in the supine and prone positions (p. 161). With improvement, 5- to 10-lb weights are added to the ankle to increase the tension. Advanced cases with functional impairment may benefit from an occupational therapy assessment.

Injection Technique An intra-articular injection should be performed under fluoroscopy.

Prognosis Most cases gradually worsen over years. Reassure the patient that surgery is very effective but should be performed in the mid-60s. Note that osteoarthritis of the hip is a gradual process. If the patient develops acute and severe pain with an abrupt change in gait, an acute process involving the hip joint needs to be excluded. Inflammatory arthritis, infective arthritis or avascular necrosis of the hip, an occult fracture in an osteoporotic femur, or malignant bony lesion of the femur should be excluded. A laboratory work-up including a complete blood count (CBC), sedimentation rate, alkaline phosphatase, and calcium are combined with bone scan, MRI scanning, and joint aspiration (as indicated) to rapidly diagnose these serious conditions.

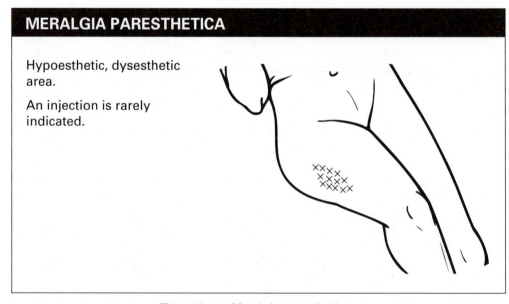

MERALGIA PARESTHETICA

Hypoesthetic, dysesthetic area.

An injection is rarely indicated.

Figure 8–4. Meralgia paresthetica.

Description Meralgia paresthetica is a compression neuropathy of the lateral femoral cutaneous nerve as the nerve exits the pelvis and the groin and enters the thigh. Obesity with an overlying panniculus, tight garments around the waist, and scar tissue near the lateral aspect of the inguinal ligament are the main causes.

Symptoms The patient has neuritic pain in a very specific area of the anterolateral thigh.

"I have this burning pain in my thigh."

"It feels funny (pointing to the outer upper thigh) when my jeans rub over the skin."

"My skin feels numb and tingly (rubbing the skin of the outer upper thigh)."

"I think I have a pinched nerve. My leg is numb right here."

Exam   Each patient should have the sensory function of the upper outer thigh examined along with a neurologic screening of the lower extremity.

EXAM SUMMARY

---

1. Hypesthesia or dysesthetic pain in the upper outer thigh
2. The lower extremity neurologic exam is normal
3. The hip, back, and sacroiliac joints are normal

---

(1) Pinprick and light touch are abnormal in a 10 × 6″ oval-shaped area on the anterolateral thigh. Note that the distribution of the lateral femoral cutaneous nerve is not strictly lateral. It is not unusual for the nerve to provide sensation to a portion of the anterior thigh! (2) The neurologic exam of the lower extremity is otherwise normal. The result of the straight leg raising is negative, and the deep tendon reflexes and distal motor strength are preserved. (3) There is no evidence of a hip, back, or sacroiliac joint abnormality.

X-Rays   Plain films of the hip and pelvis are not necessary. No characteristic changes are seen on x-ray.

Diagnosis   The diagnosis is based on the unique description of the pain, its characteristic location, the sensory abnormalities on exam, and the conspicuous absence of neurologic abnormalities in the lower leg.

Treatment   The goals of treatment are to reassure the patient that this is not a serious condition such as a pinched nerve and to recommend ways to reduce pressure over the nerve in the groin.

Step 1: Avoid tight garments.
   Discuss the need for weight loss.
   Educate the patient. "This is not a serious back problem; not a pinched nerve."

Step 2 (months): Consider carbamazepine (Tegretol) or phenytoin (Dilantin) to reduce the dysesthetic pain (advise that "This relatively minor problem should not be overtreated with harsh and potentially harmful medications!").

Step 3 (months to years): Consider a neurosurgical consultation for intractable dysesthetic cases.

Physical Therapy   Physical therapy does not play a significant role in the treatment of meralgia paresthetica. Abdominal muscle toning may reduce the pressure over the lateral femoral cutaneous nerve but is of unproven value.

Injection Technique   A local injection is not used. A nerve block adjacent to the anterior superior iliac spine can be performed by an experienced anesthesiologist.

Prognosis   Symptoms may resolve over several months depending on the presence of a reversible cause and whether or not permanent nerve damage has occurred. Surgical lysis is used in severe, unremitting cases (neurolysis). Rarely, surgical exploration of the nerve as it leaves the abdomen can be performed.

Knee

PATELLOFEMORAL DISEASES

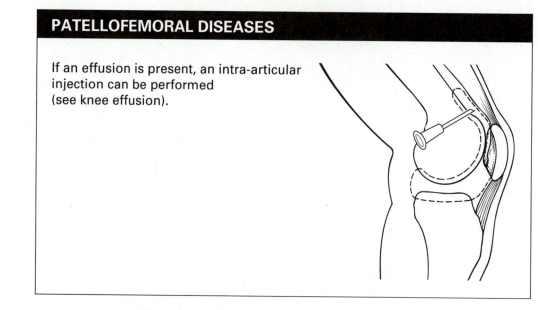

If an effusion is present, an intra-articular injection can be performed (see knee effusion).

Figure 9–1. Patellofemoral osteoarthritis injection.

Description   Several terms are used to describe the spectrum of conditions that affect the patellofemoral joint. Chondromalacia patella describes painful knee caps. Other terms, such as abnormal patellofemoral tracking, patellar subluxation, and patellofemoral arthritis describe the abnormal alignment or degenerative changes. Although some cases are due to direct trauma, most develop patellar irritation caused by abnormal alignment. Arthroscopically, the defects in the articular cartilage of the patella are focal initially (e.g., pits, cracks). Over many years, diffuse irregularities of the articular cartilage occur, (e.g., osteoarthritis). Poor muscle tone, repetitive squatting and kneeling, and direct trauma predispose to the condition.

Symptoms   The patient has knee pain (in the front of the knee), "noise" coming from the knee, or swelling.

"My knee caps ache after I run."

"I can't squat or kneel any more."

"I have this grinding sound when I bend my knee."

"Whenever I use the stairstepper or do Jazzersize, both my knees will ache that evening."

"Two years ago, I rammed my knees into the dashboard. Ever since then, my knees ache after taking long hikes through the mountains."

"I can't sit Indian style any more."

"My knees have always had this grinding noise, but now they're swelling."

Exam   Each patient should be examined for patella irritation and alignment along with an assessment of knee effusion.

EXAM SUMMARY

1. Abnormal patellofemoral tracking; abnormal Q angle
2. Painful patellar crepitation
3. Negative apprehension sign
4. Knee effusion (not common)
5. In the absence of a knee effusion, normal knee range of motion

(1) Patellofemoral tracking and alignment are assessed by inspection, by measurement of the Q angle, and by passive flexion and extension of the knee. The patella may be visibly subluxed laterally by inspection. The Q angle (the angle made by the anterior superior iliac spine, the midpatella, and the midtibial tubercle) should be less than 20 degrees. The patella may not glide smoothly in the patellofemoral groove when passively flexing and extending the knee. (2) Painful patellar crepitation is best felt by passively moving the patella back and forth across the femoral groove. The leg is placed in the extended position, and the patient is asked to relax the quadriceps muscle. With the examiner's fingers on all four poles of the patella, it is forced onto the lateral and medial femoral condyles and down into the inferior patellofemoral groove. Note that early disease may have crepitation only in the inferior portion of the groove. (3) A patellar click may be palpable over the anterior knee with passive flexion and extension. (4) The apprehension sign (pressure applied medially to laterally to cause the patella to dislocate) should be absent. (5) The presence of a knee effusion is indicative of advanced disease (p. 82). (6) In the absence of a knee effusion, uncomplicated chondromalacia should have full range of motion of the knee.

X-Rays   Three views of the knee, including the "merchant" view (Haugston view or the sunrise view), are always recommended. Films of early chondromalacia may be totally normal or show lateral subluxation on the sunrise view. As the condition progresses over many years, the patellofemoral joint space narrows, bony osteophytes form at the poles of the patella, and bony sclerosis of the patella develops.

Diagnosis   The diagnosis is based on the clinical findings of anterior knee pain associated with painful patellar crepitation. Regional anesthetic block can be helpful in differentiating the articular pain arising from the patella and a complicating periarticular process (e.g., anserine bursitis). Arthroscopy is indicated when internal derangement (meniscal tear or loose body) cannot be excluded on clinical grounds.

Treatment   The goals of treatment are to improve patellofemoral tracking, reduce pain and swelling, and retard the development of patellofemoral arthritis.

Step 1: X-ray the knee, including the merchant view.

Apply ice and elevate the knee, especially with effusion.

Avoid squatting and kneeling.

Swimming, Nordictrack, and fast walking are preferable to jogging, bicycling, and impact sports.

Straight leg-raising exercises to improve the tone of the vastus medialis obliqus. Toning will improve patellofemoral tracking (p. 161).

Step 2 (4 to 8 weeks): Reinforce exercises and restriction.

A nonsteroidal anti-inflammatory drug (NSAID) (e.g., ibuprofen [Advil, Motrin]) for 4 weeks, at full dose and at regular intervals.

Use a patellar strap (p. 180) or a Velcro patellar restraining brace (p. 181).

Step 3 (3 to 4 months): Give a local corticosteroid injection with K40 or D80 (for persistent symptoms or effusion).

Repeat the injection at 4 to 6 weeks if symptoms have not been reduced by 50%.

Step 4 (4 to 6 months): Re-emphasize the need to continue daily or thrice weekly straight leg-raising exercises.

Continue restrictions of use and motion.

Consider orthopedic referral for persistent pain and dysfunction or for cases associated with "patella alta" or Q angles greater than 20 degrees.

Physical Therapy   Physical therapy is one of the main treatments for the patellofemoral disorders.

PHYSICAL THERAPY SUMMARY

> **1.** Ice
> **2.** Straight leg raises for the quadriceps femoris and hamstring muscle toning
> **3.** Cautious use of active exercise with apparatus

ACUTELY Ice and elevation are used when symptoms are acute. *Ice* is an effective analgesic and may help to reduce swelling.

RECOVERY REHABILITATION Exercises are combined with restricted use to reduce patellofemoral irritation. *Muscle toning exercises* help to stabilize the knee joint, reduce subluxation and dislocation, and improve patellofemoral tracking. Daily straight leg raises in the supine and prone positions are performed in sets of 20 (p. 161). These exercises are performed initially without weights; however, with improvement, 5 to 10 lb weights are added at the ankle. *Active exercises,* especially on equipment, must be done with caution. Stationary bicycle exercise, rowing machines, and universal gym requiring full-knee flexion must be avoided. Fast walking, swimming, and Nordictrack-like glide machines are preferred. Exercises with limited knee flexion are preferred to exercises that move the patella back and forth in the femoral groove!

Injection Technique Exercises of the quadriceps and hamstrings are the mainstays of treatment for this condition of abnormal mechanics. Local injection has limited benefit unless persistent effusion occurs. See knee effusion for injection technique (p. 85).

Prognosis Symptomatic flares of pain or swelling can last for months. Preventative exercises cannot be overemphasized. Improvement in quadriceps and hamstring tone should retard the progression of simple chondromalacia to patellofemoral arthritis. Several surgical procedures are available, all of which attempt to correct abnormal patellofemoral tracking. Arthroscopic shaving and débridement can be combined with lateral retinacular release or tibial tubercle transposition. Surgery, like injection therapy, is not a substitute for regular quadriceps toning.

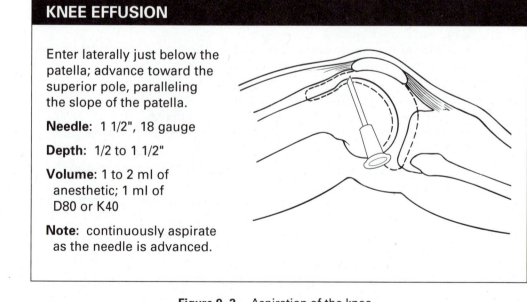

KNEE EFFUSION

Enter laterally just below the patella; advance toward the superior pole, paralleling the slope of the patella.

Needle: 1 1/2", 18 gauge

Depth: 1/2 to 1 1/2"

Volume: 1 to 2 ml of anesthetic; 1 ml of D80 or K40

Note: continuously aspirate as the needle is advanced.

Figure 9–2. Aspiration of the knee.

Description A knee effusion is an abnormal accumulation of synovial fluid. It is classified as noninflammatory or inflammatory, depending on the cellular content.

Osteoarthritis, inflammatory arthritis, chondromalacia patella, and infection (e.g., gonococcal, staphylococcal) are the most common causes. Increasing amounts of fluid interfere with the normal motion of the knee, restricting flexion first and then extension.

Symptoms   The patient complains of knee swelling, tightness in the knee, or restricted motion.

"My knee is swollen."

"I feel an egg behind my knee whenever I bend it back."

"My knee is giving out. It feels like it won't hold my weight."

"My knee feels tight."

"I have a fever inside my knee."

"My knee has become so swollen that I can't bend it back or fully straighten it."

"My right knee seems to be so much bigger than the left."

"My whole knee feels achy and tight."

"At the end of the day the swelling is so great that I limp. It feels like it's going to burst."

Exam   Maneuvers to detect knee swelling are combined with an exam of the range of motion of the knee.

EXAM SUMMARY

1. Loss of the medial and lateral peripatellar dimples
2. Synovial milking sign
3. The patellar ballottement sign
4. Suprapatellar bulging
5. Needle aspiration
6. Loss of full knee flexion

(1) With the knee in the extended position and the quadriceps muscle relaxed, the medial and lateral peripatellar dimples are inspected. Small effusions (5 to 10 ml) will fill in these normal anatomic landmarks. (2) For small effusions with high viscosity, the synovial milking sign may be positive. Pressure is held over the medial dimple (over the medial patellar retinaculum) to force the synovial fluid into the lateral compartment. When pressure is released and a milking motion is applied to the lateral dimple (over the lateral patellar retinaculum), the fluid reappears medially. Note that this test is practical only in asthenic patients. (3) The ballottement sign is positive with 10 to 15 ml of fluid. Using both hands, the synovial fluid is milked into the center of the knee from all four quadrants. With the index finger, the patella is forcibly snapped down against the femur. A moderate effusion is associated with a clicking or tapping sensation. (4) Large effusions (20 to 25 ml) fill the suprapatellar space. This area, directly below the quadriceps tendon, is usually flat or slightly concave. Large effusions cause a convexity above the superior pole of the patella. (5) Joint aspiration is the definitive test for knee effusion. This is especially true for the obese patient or for the patient with unusually large peripatellar fat pads. (6) A joint effusion should be suspected if the affected knee is enlarged and lacks full flexion. Flexion can be measured in degrees (0 degrees at full extension) or the heel-to-buttock distance can be measured. The latter is a very practical method of following the patients with knee effusions.

X-Rays   X-rays of the knee are always recommended. Plain films of the knee are used to define the extent of degenerative arthritis either at the main weightbearing joint or the patellofemoral articulation. Plain films with good soft tissue technique may provide clues to the presence of large effusions but are not a substitute for the clinical exam.

Diagnosis   A presumptive diagnosis of a knee effusion can be made on the basis of physical signs; however, a definitive diagnosis requires fluid obtained by needle aspiration. This is especially important if articular infection is suspected. Joint aspiration is mandatory whenever infection is in the differential diagnosis.

Treatment   The goals of treatment are to diagnose the underlying cause of the effusion, to reduce swelling and inflammation, and to prevent a recurrence by physical therapy exercises.

Step 1: X-ray the knee including the merchant view.
>   Aspirate the effusion for diagnostic studies (e.g., cell count and differential, crystals, glucose, Gram stain, and culture at a minimum).
>   Apply ice and elevate the knee.
>   Severe cases may require crutches with touch-down weightbearing.
>   Reduce squatting and kneeling.
>   Swimming, Nordictrack, and fast walking are preferable to jogging, bicycling, and impact sports.
>   Do straight leg raises without weights at first (p. 161).
>   A neoprene pull-on knee brace (p. 180).

Step 2 (days to 4 weeks): Reaspirate tense effusions.
>   Give a NSAID (e.g., ibuprofen [Advil, Motrin]) for 4 weeks at full dose and at regular intervals.

Step 3 (3 to 6 weeks): Reaspirate and inject with D80 or K40.
>   Repeat the injection at 4 to 6 weeks if symptoms are not reduced by 50%.
>   Re-emphasize straight leg-raising exercises with ankle weights.

Step 4 (2 to 4 months): Take another x-ray or magnetic resonance imaging (MRI) scan or do arthrography for persistent effusions (especially those associated with mechanical symptoms).
>   Consider orthopedic consultation, depending on the underlying cause (e.g., meniscal tears, loose bodies, advanced osteoarthritis).

Physical Therapy   Physical therapy plays an essential role in the active treatment and prevention of knee effusions.

PHYSICAL THERAPY SUMMARY

> 1. Apply ice and elevate the knee
> 2. Crutches, touch-down weightbearing
> 3. Straight leg raises
> 4. Active exercises with caution

ACUTELY   For the first few days apply ice, elevate the knee, and restrict weightbearing. *Ice* and elevation are always recommended for acute knee effusions. An ice bag, a bag of frozen corn, or an iced towel from the freezer applied for 10 to 15 minutes is effective for swelling and analgesia. *Crutches,* a *walker,* or a *cane* may be necessary in the first few days.

RECOVERY/REHABILITATION   After the acute symptoms subside, toning exercises are combined with restricted use. *Straight leg-raising exercises* are always recommended to restore muscular support (p. 161). Initially, these are performed without weights in sets of 20, with each held 5 seconds. With improvement in strength, a 5- to 10-lb weight is added to the ankle. These exercises are performed in the prone and supine positions to tone the quadriceps femoris and hamstring muscles. *Active exercises*, especially on equipment, must be used with caution. Exercise on a stationary bicycle, a rowing machine, or a universal gym may be irritating to a distended joint. Fast walking, swimming, Nordic track-like glide machines, and other limited impact exercises requiring much less flexion are preferred.

Injection Technique   Aspiration and injection of the knee has variable results, depending on the underlying cause. Any knee that has a significant effusion should be "tapped" for diagnostic studies. Moderate-to-severe inflammatory conditions can be treated with intra-articular corticosteroids, often with dramatic results.

Position: The patient is placed in the supine position with the leg fully extended.

Technique: A lateral approach is easiest and safest. The patella is gently subluxed laterally. The lateral edge of the patella is palpated, and skin anesthesia is performed ½" below it at the midpoint. The needle is then directed toward the superior pole of the patella and is advanced gently down to the tissue resistance of the lateral retinaculum. An additional ½ to 1 ml of anesthesia is placed here, just outside the synovial lining. The needle is withdrawn. Next, an 18-gauge 1½" needle attached to a 20-ml syringe is advanced down to the retinaculum and then into the joint (a giving way sensation or pop is often felt along with discomfort). The bevel of the needle is rotated 180 degrees, and complete aspiration is attempted. Gentle pressure against the medial retinaculum and joint line may facilitate aspiration.

If the fluid is relatively clear (the examiner should be able to read newsprint through a low cell count fluid), either 1 ml of K40 or D80 is injected using the same 18-gauge needle left in place.

Restrictions: The patient is instructed to limit activities for 3 days and to follow the aforementioned restrictions for the next 30 days. Quadriceps and hamstring exercises are resumed on day 4.

Prognosis   The response to aspiration and injection depends on the underlying cause. Mild to moderate inflammatory effusions (cell counts from 1000 to 20,000) respond most dramatically, with months of relief. The response with bland effusion (cell counts in the 100s) is less predictable. Poor responses to intra-articular steroids suggest either a noninflammatory process or a mechanical process (more likely surgical). The latter cases should be evaluated further with another x-ray, MRI scanning, or arthroscopy. Synovectomy is reserved for treatment failures, and is most often performed on patients with rheumatoid arthritis.

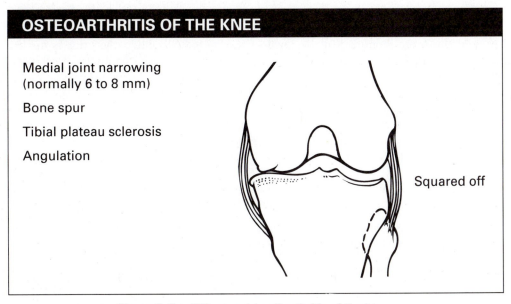

OSTEOARTHRITIS OF THE KNEE

Medial joint narrowing
(normally 6 to 8 mm)

Bone spur

Tibial plateau sclerosis

Angulation

Squared off

Figure 9–3.   "Wear and tear" arthritis of the knee.

Description   Osteoarthritis of the knee is a wear-and-tear, noninflammatory arthritis that affects the three compartments of joint (the medial, lateral, and patellofemoral joint). A family history, obesity, genu valgum and genu varum, previous meniscectomy, and previous fractures of the distal femur and proximal tibia predispose to this condition. Pathologically, there is asymmetric wear of the articular cartilage, bony osteophyte formation, and sclerosis of the subchondral bone and in advanced cases subchondral cyst formation.

Symptoms   The patient has knee pain, knee swelling, or deformity.

''My knee gets stiff and painful at the end of the day.''

''I can't do my 'folks walks' anymore . . . my knees ache so bad.''

''My knees make this awful sound every time I kneel down to pray in church.''

''I'm too embarrassed to wear dresses anymore . . . my knees look so bony.''

''My knees have ached for a long time . . . now they swell really badly and they give out all the time . . . I'm afraid to even go to the store.''

''I can't bend my knees any more.''

''When I was 22, I had my cartilage removed from my right knee. It swelled and popped a lot then. Now the whole thing just aches.''

Exam   Each patient should be examined for the presence of an effusion, loss of range of motion, and loss of smooth mechanical function.

EXAM SUMMARY

1. Joint line tenderness, medially greater than laterally
2. Crepitation with passive and active motion
3. Palpable bony osteophytes
4. Knee effusion
5. Loss of full flexion or full extension
6. Loss of smooth mechanical motion

(1) Tenderness is present at the joint line, more commonly on the medial side. The joint lines are identified at the level of the midpatella when the knee is in the extended position and the quadriceps muscle is relaxed. (2) The hallmark of osteoarthritis is crepitation of the knee, palpable at the joint line when the knee is passively flexed and extended. This is in contrast to the crepitation felt anteriorly seen with chondromalacia. (3) Advanced cases have palpable bony osteophytes at the joint line. The enlargement is greatest at the medial tibial plateau. (4) Knee effusions commonly complicate osteoarthritis. Effusions that develop acutely and knee effusions over 20 to 25 ml interfere with full flexion. (5) As the condition progresses, the bony osteophytes and the damage to the articular cartilage interfere with full range of motion. (6) Occasionally, an acute change in the mechanical function of the knee occurs. Popping, locking, or other mechanical symptoms may suggest a ''degenerative meniscal tear.''

X-Rays   X-rays of the knee (posteroanterior, lateral, and merchant views) are always recommended. Plain films of the knee provide an accurate diagnosis as well as a prognosis. The distance between the medial tibial plateau and the medial femoral condyle is normally 6 to 8 mm. As the condition progresses, this space gradually narrows. Serial measurements can be used to predict when surgical consultation is necessary. If mechanical symptoms outweigh the clinical findings, MRI scanning is obtained to evaluate for a degenerative meniscus or a loose body.

Diagnosis A presumptive clinical diagnosis, based on knee pain, crepitation, bony enlargement, and swelling can be confirmed by plain films of the knee. A regional anesthetic block can be used to differentiate the pain arising from the joint from the pain arising from the periarticular structures.

Treatment The goals of treatment are to relieve pain, treat the accompanying effusion, and preserve function and stage for surgery.

Step 1: X-ray both knees in the standing position (measure the cartilage remaining).

> Advise on weight loss.
> Suggest padded insoles and supportive shoes (p. 185).
> Limit squatting, kneeling, and repetitious impact sports.
> Encourage swimming, cross-country skiing, Nordic track, etc.
> Recommend daily straight leg raises with weights (p. 161).
> Recommend heat in the morning and ice for swelling after activities.
> Prescribe a NSAID (e.g., ibuprofen [Advil, Motrin]) in full dose and at regular intervals for 4 weeks.

Step 2 (weeks to months): If symptoms are persistent, prescribe a 3- to 4-week course of a NSAID from a different chemical class or a local injection for persistent effusion.

> Repeat in 4 to 6 weeks if symptoms are not reduced by 50%.
> No more than three or four injections should be given each year.

Step 3 (months to years): X-ray again for progressive symptoms.

> Consider either a Velcro patellar restraining brace or a more rigid metal-hinged derotational brace (p. 181).
> Consider an orthopedic referral for patients who do not have any medical contraindication for surgery if (1) pain is intractable, (2) function is severely compromised, (3) 80 to 90% of the articular cartilage has worn away, or (4) progressive angulation has occurred.

Physical Therapy Physical therapy plays an important role in the overall treatment and management of patients with osteoarthritis. General care of the knee is recommended with emphasis on toning the quadriceps and hamstring muscles by straight leg-raising exercises (pp. 159 to 161).

Injection Technique A local injection can provide dramatic short-term relief (see Knee Effusion p. 82). It is usually reserved for those with advanced disease who either cannot have surgery or who need to postpone surgery because of age or convenience. Note that a lateral approach for aspiration and injection (p. 85) may not be suitable for all patients, especially those with severe hypertrophic patellofemoral disease. In these cases, a medial approach can be performed that is analogous to the lateral approach, except that the point of entry is at the intersection of the medial edge and the midpoint of the patella.

Prognosis Osteoarthritis of the knee is a relentlessly progressive problem that is characterized by periodic flares of pain and swelling. Medication either by mouth or by injection should be reserved for these exacerbations. Dramatic changes in clinical findings or rapid progression of wear may reflect a degenerative meniscal tear, the effects of increased angulation, underlying rheumatic disease, or a complicating infection. Take another x-ray. A synovial fluid analysis or an MRI of the knee may be necessary. Surgery is indicated for advanced disease. Arthroplasty is the surgery of choice in patients 60 to 65 years of age. Wedge osteotomy of the tibia is a reasonable option for younger patients.

PREPATELLAR BURSITIS

The bursa is entered at the base and parallel to the patella; the needle is passed into the center of the sac.

Needle: 1 1/2", 18 gauge

Depth: 1/4"

Volume: 1 ml of anesthetic; 1 ml of K40

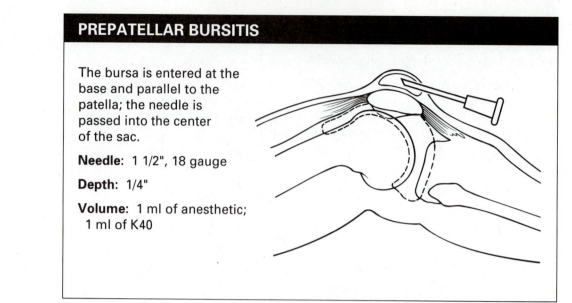

Figure 9–4. Prepatellar bursa aspiration.

Description   Prepatellar bursitis is an inflammation of the bursal sac located between the patella and the overlying skin. Its common name is housemaid's knee. Repetitive pressure, gout, and staphylococcal infection are the three common causes.

Symptoms   The patient has knee swelling and knee pain just over the patella.

"My knee is swollen."

"I'm a housekeeper. I have to work on my knees a lot. Even though I am careful and wear knee pads, my right knee has begun to swell."

"My knee is inflamed."

"I have a bump over my knee cap."

"It feels like a bunch of little marbles just under the skin."

"I bumped my knee against the kitchen cabinet and within hours it had swollen up."

Exam   Each patient should be examined for the degree of swelling and inflammation over the patella along with an estimation of the amount of fluid.

EXAM SUMMARY

1. Swelling and inflammation directly over the patella
2. Bursal sac tenderness versus bursal sac thickening
3. Normal range of motion of the knee

(1) A cystic collection of fluid is palpable directly over the patella. Inflammatory signs are variable depending on the cause of symptoms and amount of time they have occurred. (2) Tenderness is present over the entire sac in acute cases. Tenderness is absent in 10% of cases that have developed chronic cobblestone-like thickening. (3) The range of motion of the knee is normal in an uncomplicated case. The extra-articular fluid does not interfere with motion, as opposed to the limitation of flexion that occurs with a large knee effusion or an effusion that develops acutely!

X-Rays X-rays of the knee are not necessary for the diagnosis. Plain films of the knee show the soft tissue swelling above the patella on the lateral views. Note that calcification in the quadriceps tendon at the superior pole of the patella is not related to this condition. This is a tendon calcification that commonly occurs and does not indicate disease.

Diagnosis The diagnosis is suggested by the presence of swelling and inflammation over the patella and is confirmed by simple aspiration.

Treatment The goals of treatment are to identify the cause of the swelling, to reduce swelling and inflammation, to encourage the walls of the bursa to readhere, and to prevent chronic bursitis.

Step 1: Aspirate the bursa for diagnostic studies: Gram stain and culture, crystals, and hematocrit.

Apply a compression dressing for 24 to 36 hours after aspiration.

Avoid direct pressure.

A neoprene pull-on knee brace (p. 180) or Velcro knee pads (p. 180).

An NSAID (e.g., Advil, Motrin) may be helpful.

Step 2 (1 to 2 days): Give an antibiotic for infection, do an evaluation and treatment for gout, or do a reaspiration and injection with K40.

Continue padding and protection.

Educate the patient, "Ten to 15% remain swollen or thickened regardless of treatment."

Step 3 (4 to 6 weeks): Reaspirate and inject with K40 if symptoms have not been reduced by 50%.

Squatting and kneeling may have to be limited.

Step 4 (months): Consider an orthopedic consultation for a bursectomy.

Physical Therapy Physical therapy does not play a significant role in the treatment of prepatellar bursitis. General care of the knee is recommended with emphasis on toning the quadriceps and hamstring muscles by straight leg-raising exercises.

Injection Technique Aspiration and injection is the treatment of choice. All bursae should be aspirated to determine the cause. Aspiration and injection with K40 will effectively treat 85% of cases.

Position: The patient is placed in the supine position with the leg fully extended.

Technique: The base of the bursa is identified. The skin and subcutaneous tissue are anesthetized using a 25-gauge needle. Then, an 18-gauge needle attached to a 10-ml syringe is passed into the center of the sac, paralleling the patella. The needle is rotated 180 degrees so that the bevel is down. The fluid is aspirated completely, and with the needle in place a corticosteroid is injected. A pressure dressing is applied using gauze and Elastoplast.

Restrictions: Avoid repetitious bending and kneeling for the next 30 days.

A pull-on knee brace may be helpful.

Prognosis Fifty to 60% of cases will either spontaneously resolve or respond to simple aspiration. The remaining cases will require one or two local injections of K40. Five to 10% of cases fail conservative care and show persistent swelling. These can be referred for definitive bursectomy. An additional 5% of cases will have persistent bursal sac thickening and chronic bursitis. Surgical treatment of these cases is individualized. Note that this bursal sac does not interfere with the normal function of the knee. Persistent swelling or thickening of the bursal sac alone is not an indication for surgery. Patients troubled with persistent pain and irritation from repetitive kneeling (e.g., carpet layers, cement finishers) should be considered for surgery.

ANSERINE BURSITIS

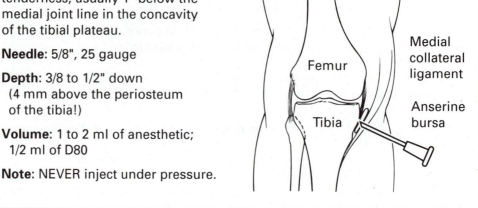

Enter over the point of maximum tenderness, usually 1" below the medial joint line in the concavity of the tibial plateau.

Needle: 5/8", 25 gauge

Depth: 3/8 to 1/2" down (4 mm above the periosteum of the tibia!)

Volume: 1 to 2 ml of anesthetic; 1/2 ml of D80

Note: NEVER inject under pressure.

Figure 9–5. Anserine bursa injection.

Description   Anserine bursitis is an inflammation of the bursal sac located between the medial tibial plateau/medial collateral ligament and the conjoined tendon formed by the gracilis, sartorius, and semitendinosus tendons. It becomes inflamed as a result of osteoarthritis of the knee or knee effusion or from any disturbance of gait. With the exception of direct trauma, it is usually caused by another lower extremity musculoskeletal process.

Symptoms   The patient has knee pain that is often localized to a well-defined area of the inner knee.

"I have a very sharp knee pain right here (pointing to the inner aspect of the knee)."

"I can't sleep on my side. When my knees touch, I get this really sharp pain on the inside of my knee."

"I don't know what happened. I didn't have an injury. I slowly developed this sharp pain inside my knee."

"The inside of my knee looks a little swollen and is very tender to the touch."

"I sleep with a pillow between my legs because my knee is tender."

"I was hit with a line drive when I was playing baseball. The ball hit me in the inside of my knee. The pain was so sharp I couldn't walk for several days."

Exam   Each patient should be examined for a well-localized area of irritation at the medial tibial plateau along with a thorough exam of the knee and gait.

EXAM SUMMARY

1. Local tenderness 1¼" below the medial joint line
2. Negative result on valgus stress testing of the medial collateral ligament
3. Abnormalities of the knee joint or of the gait
4. Regional anesthetic block to confirm the diagnosis

(1) Local tenderness is present 1 to 1¼" below the medial joint line. The quarter-sized area is located in the midline of the medial tibial plateau. (2) Valgus stress testing

of the knee does not aggravate the pain—that is, the signs of a medial collateral ligament strain are absent! (3) The knee and lower extremities are examined for any primary musculoskeletal process.

X-Rays   X-rays of the knee are not necessary for the diagnosis. Plain films of the knee are normal for an uncomplicated case of anserine bursitis. Plain films, arthrocentesis, or MRI scanning are used to evaluate for a primary cause.

Diagnosis   The diagnosis is based on the localized medial tibial plateau tenderness, the absence of signs indicating a medial collateral ligament strain, and pain relief with local anesthetic. A regional anesthetic block in the bursa is used to differentiate the pain of osteoarthritis of the medial compartment, the pain of chondromalacia patella, and the pain from a tear of the medial meniscus.

Treatment   The goals of treatment are to reduce the pain and swelling in the bursa and to identify and treat any underlying cause.

Step 1: X-ray the knee including the merchant view.

Evaluate for underlying causes (e.g., knee effusion, gait disturbance, internal derangement).

Eliminate squatting and minimize direct pressure (pillow between the knees at night).

Avoid crossing of the legs.

Limit repetitive bending.

Apply ice.

An NSAID (e.g., ibuprofen [Advil, Motrin]) may be helpful.

Step 2 (6 to 8 weeks): Give an injection of D80.

Give another injection of D80 in 4 to 6 weeks if symptoms and signs have not been reduced by 50%.

Continue to evaluate for secondary causes.

Step 3 (8 to 10 weeks): Do straight leg raises with weights (p. 161).

Take care when squatting, kneeling, and doing repetitive knee flexion.

Physical Therapy   Physical therapy does not play a significant role in the treatment of anserine bursitis.

PHYSICAL THERAPY SUMMARY

> **1.** Ice
> **2.** Phonophoresis for temporary relief
> **3.** General care of the knee (p. 160)

Ice over the bursa will effectively control pain and some of the swelling. *Phonophoresis* of a hydrocortisone gel may provide temporary relief. *General care of the knee* is recommended with emphasis on toning the quadriceps femoris and the hamstring muscles by straight leg raising exercises (pp. 159 to 161).

Injection Technique   Any underlying condition should be evaluated and treated before treating the bursa primarily. If no underlying cause is found or if symptoms persist for more than 6 weeks, corticosteroid injection is recommended.

Position: The patient is placed in the supine position with the leg extended. The patient is asked to relax the thigh muscles.

Technique: The point of maximum tenderness is palpated over the concavity of the tibial plateau. Typically, this is in the midline 1″ below the medial joint line of the knee. The needle is inserted at this site, advanced down to the bone, and withdrawn 4 mm. This is to ensure placement above the medial collateral ligament. If the local tenderness is significantly decreased, then ½ ml of D80 is injected. The medication is massaged in for 5 minutes.

Restriction: Walking, jogging, and stair climbing are restricted for 3 days and limited for 30 days. Bracing is not necessary except for any underlying condition.

Prognosis   Persistent symptoms or a recurrence is more likely if there is an underlying cause. Injection is otherwise very successful in controlling local symptoms. Bursectomy is not advised.

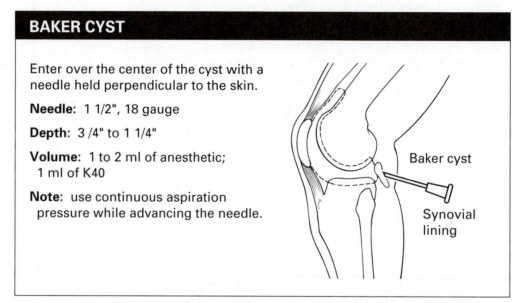

BAKER CYST

Enter over the center of the cyst with a needle held perpendicular to the skin.

Needle: 1 1/2", 18 gauge

Depth: 3 /4" to 1 1/4"

Volume: 1 to 2 ml of anesthetic; 1 ml of K40

Note: use continuous aspiration pressure while advancing the needle.

Baker cyst

Synovial lining

Figure 9–6.   Baker cyst decompression and injection.

Description   A Baker cyst is an abnormal collection of synovial fluid in the popliteal fossa. It must be distinguished from the more common semimembranosus bursa, which is an evagination of the synovial lining of the knee. Both are located on the medial side of the popliteal fossa, and both are caused by an overproduction of synovial fluid. However, only the Baker cyst is a separate anatomic structure. Fluid escaping the normal confines of the synovial lining causes a fibrous reaction in the subcutaneous tissue and cyst formation.

Symptoms   The patient has tightness behind the knee or pain down the back of the leg.

"My doctor told me that I have a cyst behind my knee."

"I felt a lump behind my knee."

"When I bend my knee back, it feels like an egg is behind my knee."

"My knee seems swollen and tight."

"My regular doctor told me I have bad circulation. The doctor in the emergency room thought I had a blood clot in my leg. I'm really confused. I've had all these tests and I still don't know why I have this pain in my leg."

Exam   Each patient should be examined for a palpable, cystic mass in the medial aspect of the popliteal fossa.

EXAM SUMMARY

> 1. A cystic mass in the popliteal fossa
> 2. Impaired knee flexion
> 3. Chronic knee effusion
> 4. No evidence of peripheral vascular insufficiency or deep venous thrombosis

(1) With the patient in the prone position and the leg fully extended, an oblong, cystic mass is visible and palpable in the medial popliteal fossa. (2) Large cysts may impair knee flexion by as much as 10 to 15 degrees. (3) Signs of a knee effusion may be present (p. 83). (4) Signs of vascular insufficiency (suggesting a popliteal aneurysm) and signs of deep venous thrombosis of popliteal veins (pain in the posterior calf) are absent.

X-Rays   X-rays of the knee are not necessary for the diagnosis. Plain films of the popliteal fossa are normal. Films of the knee may show changes of osteoarthritis or rheumatoid arthritis (primary causes). Ultrasound can be used to define the size and extent of the cyst. Arthrography may reveal a sinus tract from the synovial cavity to the cyst.

Diagnosis   A tentative diagnosis is based on the presence of a palpable, popliteal mass or by the demonstration of a fluid-filled cyst on ultrasonography. A definitive diagnosis, however, requires aspiration of the characteristic clear, nonbloody, highly tenacious fluid.

Treatment   The goals of treatment are to decompress the abnormal accumulation of fluid, to correct any underlying cause of chronic knee effusion, and to determine the need for surgery.

Step 1: Observe (some spontaneously resolve!).

> Evaluate and treat any underlying cause of chronic knee effusion (e.g., rheumatoid arthritis, degenerative arthritis).
>
> Restrict squatting, kneeling, and repetitious bending.
>
> Encourage straight leg-raising exercises with weights (p. 161).
>
> Consider a neoprene pull-on knee brace (p. 180).

Step 2 (4 to 6 weeks): Perform a simple cyst aspiration (remove as much fluid as possible).

> Continue use of the neoprene brace (p. 180).
>
> Educate the patient, "These types of cysts frequently recur regardless of which treatment is used."

Step 3 (8 to 10 weeks): Aspirate and inject with K40.

> Repeat the injection in 4 to 6 weeks if the size of the cyst has not decreased by 50%.

Step 4 (3 to 6 months): If improved, do straight leg-raising exercises with weights (p. 161).

> Avoid repetitive flexion and squatting.
>
> Consider surgical removal if the patient is a surgical candidate, if all causes of excessive fluid production have been treated optimally, and if the cyst is interfering with the normal function of the knee.

Physical Therapy   Physical therapy plays a minor role in the treatment of a Baker cyst. General care of the knee is recommended with emphasis on toning the quadriceps femoris and hamstring muscles by straight leg-raising exercises (pp. 159 to 161).

Injection Technique   Simple aspiration with or without injection of corticosteroids is the preferred treatment.

Position: The patient is placed in the prone position with the leg extended.

Technique: The skin directly over the cyst is anesthetized with a 25-gauge needle. An 18-gauge needle that is attached to a 20-ml syringe is held vertically and passed down into the center of the cyst. The outer wall is often felt as giving way or pop at approximately ¾ to 1 ¼" down. Continuous aspiration pressure is used while advancing. After the cyst is entered, the needle is cautiously advanced until the tissue resistance of the back wall is felt or fluid can no longer be easily aspirated. The needle is then withdrawn ⅛ to ⅜". This is to ensure that the needle remains in the cavity as the fluid is removed. Manual pressure is applied to either side of the needle to assist in fluid recovery. With the needle left in place, 1 ml of K40 is injected into the cyst.

Restriction: The patient is instructed to avoid squatting, and excessive bending for the next 3 days and to limit these for the ensuing 30 days.

Prognosis   Aspiration and injection with corticosteroids can provide symptomatic relief for months. Like all ganglions, however, the recurrence rate is high, especially if an underlying chronic knee effusion is present. Persistent cases can be referred for surgical removal. Unfortunately, as with medical therapy, recurrence does occur after surgery.

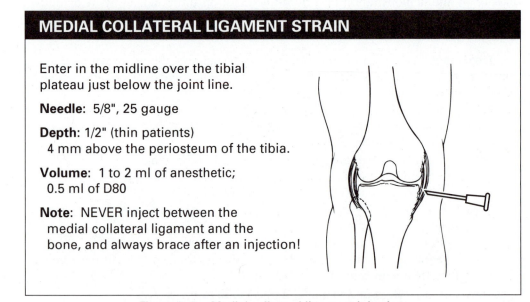

MEDIAL COLLATERAL LIGAMENT STRAIN

Enter in the midline over the tibial plateau just below the joint line.

Needle: 5/8", 25 gauge

Depth: 1/2" (thin patients)
4 mm above the periosteum of the tibia.

Volume: 1 to 2 ml of anesthetic;
0.5 ml of D80

Note: NEVER inject between the medial collateral ligament and the bone, and always brace after an injection!

Figure 9–7.   Medial collateral ligament injection.

Description   A medial collateral ligament strain is an irritation, inflammation, or partial separation of the inner "hinge" ligament of the knee. Strains are classified as first, second, or third degree on the basis of the amount of motion on valgus stress testing. Ligaments that are irritated and inflamed but otherwise intact are classified as first-degree strains. Ligaments that are partially torn are classified as second-degree separations. Ligaments that are completely disrupted with gross instability of the knee are classified as third-degree separations.

Symptoms   The patient has knee pain along the inner aspect of the knee joint and has difficulty with walking, pivoting, and twisting.

"I was playing touch football, and I was tackled from the right side causing immediate pain along the inner part of my knee."

"I was getting out of the bathtub when my leg caught, my body twisted, and my leg was wrenched. Ever since, I have had pain and sensitivity along the inside of my knee."

"I sprained my knee when I tripped on the rug."

"Every time I twist my leg, I get this sharp pain along the side of my knee."

"I can't even turn over in bed. My leg gets snagged up in the sheets, and any amount of twisting just kills me."

"My knee has been swollen for months, but now it feels different. It feels loose and sloppy."

Exam   Each patient should be examined for the degree of irritation, inflammation, and laxity of the medial collateral ligament along with a general assessment of the stability of the knee.

EXAM SUMMARY

1. Local tenderness at the medial joint line down to the insertion on the tibia
2. Pain aggravated by valgus stress testing
3. Laxity of the medial joint compartment
4. Associated knee effusion, anterior cruciate ligament tear, or medial meniscal tear

(1) Tenderness is located from the medial joint line down to the insertion of the medial collateral ligament on the tibial plateau. The tenderness is usually about 1" long, paralleling the length of the ligament. (2) Valgus stress testing, applied with the leg in the extended position, causes acute pain and (3) may demonstrate laxity of the medial structures. Significant medial collateral ligament strain may also be aggravated by forcibly externally rotating the tibia on the femur with the knee bent at 90 degrees. (4) The remaining examination of the knee may show effusion, laxity, or disruption of the anterior cruciate ligament or a medial meniscal tear. Trauma severe enough to cause a third-degree separation is often enough to disrupt other supporting tissues of the knee.

X-Rays   X-rays are not necessary for the diagnosis. Routine plain films of the knee are usually normal. Avulsion fractures are unusual. Calcification of the ligament can occur months to years later. A 1 to 1¼" crescent-shaped calcification along the medial joint line is referred to as Pellegrini-Stieda syndrome. This radiographic finding is unique but does not correlate directly with clinically findings!

Diagnosis   The diagnosis is based on a history of a "line of pain" crossing the medial joint line and on an exam showing local medial knee tenderness that is consistently aggravated by valgus stress testing. A regional anesthetic block is rarely used to differentiate this local periarticular process from an intra-articular condition.

Treatment   The goals of treatment are to allow the ligament to reattach to its bony origins, to strengthen the muscular support to the knee, and to avoid activities that would reinjure the ligament.

Step 1: Advise crutches for the first 7 days of an acute injury!

A Velcro knee immobilizer with metal stays or a Velcro straight leg brace should be worn continuously (p. 181).

Apply ice at the joint line.

An NSAID (e.g., ibuprofen [Advil, Motrin]) may help to control the pain.

Activities of daily living for the first 2 to 4 weeks should not include sports!

Step 2 (2 to 4 weeks): Do straight leg raises without weight (after the pain resolves).

Continue bracing with activities.

Educate the patient, "These ligament injuries can take months to heal."

Step 3 (6 to 8 weeks): Give a local injection of D80 coupled with continuous bracing for 4 weeks.

Gradually resume activities.

Do straight leg raises with weights.

Brace during sports, and avoid pivoting and twisting.

Physical Therapy   Physical therapy plays a minor role in the active treatment of medial collateral ligament strains but a major role in rehabilitation.

PHYSICAL THERAPY SUMMARY

1. Ice
2. Straight leg-raising exercises without weights (while wearing the knee brace)
3. Straight leg-raising exercises with weights for rehabilitation
4. Cautious use of exercise equipment

ACUTELY   Ice, elevation, crutches, and limited use are advised in the first 7 to 14 days. Application of *ice* over the medial tibial plateau is an effective local analgesic. It is combined with restricted use to control the acute symptoms and to allow the injured ligament to reattach to the bone.

RECOVERY   After 7 to 10 days, exercises are begun to strengthen the supporting structures of the knee. While still wearing the knee brace, *straight leg-raising exercises* are performed without additional weight (p. 161). The leg is kept perfectly straight to avoid placing torque on the ligament.

REHABILITATION   As the ligament strengthens, *weighted straight leg-raising exercises* can be started to enhance the toning of the quadriceps and hamstring muscles (p. 161). *Active exercises*, especially on equipment, must be done with caution. A knee brace should be worn. Exercises and equipment that twist the knee or require pivoting must be avoided. Fast walking, swimming (kicking with the legs straight), and the Nordictrack-like equipment are preferred.

Injection Technique   Immobilization and time are the treatments of choice. When the ligament fails to improve after many weeks, local injection is recommended (but only with concurrent immobilization).

Position: The patient is placed in the supine position with the leg fully extended.

Technique: The tibial plateau is identified, just below the medial joint line. A 25-gauge needle is inserted and advanced down to the periosteum of the tibia while held perpendicular to the skin. Once the bone has been touched, the needle is withdrawn 4 mm to ensure that the injection is above the medial collateral ligament attachment. (Err on the superficial side rather than too deep; deep injections may lift the ligament off the bone.) After local anesthesia, retest for local tenderness and aggravation with valgus stress testing. If these are greatly improved, inject the same area with ½ ml of D80. Massage the medication in for 5 minutes.

Restrictions: Absolutely restrict twisting, squatting, and kneeling for the next 30 days. Continue to wear the knee immobilizer.

Prognosis   This injury can take months to heal. Recurrent strain depends on whether the ligament is able to reattach to its normal bony insertion or whether irreparable tissue damage has occurred. Recurrent cases should be managed with immobilization, either a Velcro brace or a rigid metal brace. Surgical reconstruction is not advised unless the anterior cruciate ligament is damaged concurrently and the knee is unstable.

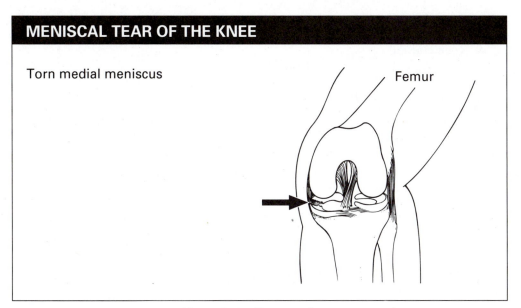

MENISCAL TEAR OF THE KNEE

Torn medial meniscus

Femur

Figure 9–8. Torn meniscus.

Description   A torn meniscus is a disruption of the fibrocartilage pads located between the femoral condyles and the tibial plateaus. Tears are classified as partial or complex; anterior, lateral, or posterior; traumatic or degenerative; or horizontal, vertical, radial, parrot beak, or bucket-handle. Because of their strategic location and inherent shock-absorbing properties, significant tears lead to loss of smooth motion of the knee and osteoarthritis after many years.

Symptoms   The patient complains of "popping, locking, and giving out" or a vague sense that the knee is not moving properly.

"My knee locks up whenever I get it in a certain bent position."

"My knee catches."

"My knee locks up on me when I bend down. When I stand up, it won't straighten right away. When it pops, I feel a bunch of pain and then it releases. It's always right here (pointing to the inner knee)."

"I can't squat anymore."

"If I twist just right, I get this real sharp pain."

"I was getting out of the car. My leg was twisted. I tried to shift my weight when I felt this loud pop and immediate sharp pain inside my knee."

"I can't put my finger on it, but whenever I try to shift my weight, the pain inside my knee practically kills me."

Exam   Each patient should be examined for loss of smooth mechanical function, for the presence of a joint effusion, and for specific meniscal signs.

EXAM SUMMARY

1. The exam result may be normal
2. General function of the knee: flexion and extension, active squatting, "duck waddle"
3. A positive McMurry sign or Apley grinding sign
4. Knee effusion
5. Underlying signs of osteoarthritis

(1) Patients with certain types of meniscal tears can have a completely normal knee exam. Partial tears, horizontal tears, and anterior tears may not produce abnormal knee signs because of their size and sequestered locations. These types of tears do not interfere with the normal mechanics of the knee and thus are less significant clinically! (2) Screening tests for significant meniscal tears should start with an assessment of general knee function. The knee can be assessed by observing gait, passive and active flexion and extension, squatting, and duck waddling. The latter is virtually impossible with large, complex, vertical, or bucket-handle tears. (3) The McMurry test and the Apley grinding test are relatively specific for meniscal tears; however, their sensitivity is poor. These tests have a false-negative rate of 20%. The McMurry maneuver should be performed several times. The knee is fully flexed. The tibia is rotated internally (relative to the femur) to trap the lateral meniscus and externally to trap the medial meniscus. A popping sensation under the examiner's fingers held firmly along the joint line is considered abnormal. (4) Large or complex tears and tears associated with degenerative arthritis often have a joint effusion. Signs of underlying osteoarthritis may be present, either as a cause of the degenerative meniscus or as a result of a long-standing meniscal tear!

X-Rays   X-rays of the knee, including the merchant, tunnel, posteroanterior, and lateral views, are recommended. Plain films of the knee may show degenerative change, calcification of the meniscus, or calcified loose bodies. The tunnel view demonstrates the intercondylar notch and may show a sequestered loose body! MRI scanning will define the extent and the type of meniscal tear. Note that MRI scanning must be interpreted cautiously. The images obtained from MRI provide information that may or may not be clinically useful. Mucinoid degenerative change of the meniscus is frequently seen and is a normal part of the aging process. This should not be interpreted as a torn meniscus. Arthroscopy is the definitive diagnostic and therapeutic test for a clinically significant meniscal tear!

Diagnosis   A tentative diagnosis is based on the history of mechanical catching or locking along with corroborative signs on exam. The diagnosis is confirmed either by MRI scanning or by arthroscopy. Note that the decision to proceed to MRI or arthroscopy should be based on the patient's age, the patient's operative candidacy, and the need to proceed with surgery. The surgical decision should be based on the type of tear, its location, the likelihood that leaving it in might lead to articular cartilage damage, and the frequency of symptoms!

Treatment   The goals of treatment are to define the type and extent of the tear, to strengthen the muscular support of the knee, and to determine the need for surgery.

Step 1: Rest, stop sports, and restrict squatting, kneeling, and repetitious bending. Apply ice and elevate the knee.
Crutches may be necessary for acute symptoms.

Straight leg-raising exercises without weights are begun as the pain begins to wane (p. 161)

A neoprene pull-on knee brace may afford some protection (p. 180).

NSAIDs (e.g., ibuprofen [Advil, Motrin]) may help with pain relief.

Step 2 (2 to 4 weeks): Aspirate persistent knee effusions for diagnostic studies and to relieve pain. Do an MRI scan if mechanical symptoms and effusion persist.

Step 3 (4 to 6 weeks): Consider an orthopedic consultation for persistent effusion and frequent, disabling symptoms.

Educate the patient, "Arthritis can result if severely damaged cartilage remains in the joint. Unfortunately, removal of a large part of the 'shock absorber' cartilage may lead to premature arthritis."

Straight leg-raising exercises with weights are continued.

Physical Therapy   Physical therapy does not play a significant role in the active treatment of a surgical meniscal tear but is very important in the preoperative preparation and the postoperative rehabilitation process. *General care of the knee* is always recommended with particular emphasis on strengthening the quadriceps and hamstring muscles that have been weakened by disuse (p. 159). For nonsurgical meniscal tears, even greater emphasis is placed on toning the thigh muscles. *Toning exercises* provide greater stability to the knee, allow the joint surfaces to better approximate, and increase the knee's endurance. These combine to reduce the knee's susceptibility to injury.

Injection Technique   Aspiration of tense, bloody effusions are recommended. Local corticosteroid injections are helpful in the select group with degenerative arthritis complicated by a degenerative meniscus. The mainstay of treatment is basic knee care or surgery if symptoms demand it (see Knee Effusion for the technique of knee aspiration on p. 85).

Prognosis   The management of meniscal tears depends on the type of tear (e.g., intrasubstance, horizontal, or vertical), the presence of significant "mechanical" symptoms, and the presence of persistent knee effusion. Intrasubstance and horizontal tears can be managed medically with rest, restriction, exercises, and aspiration. Vertical tears (in contact with articular cartilage); tears associated with large, persistent effusions; and tears with frequently disabling symptoms should be evaluated by arthroscopy. Partial or complete meniscectomy is determined at the time of operation.

CHAPTER 10

Ankle and Foot

ANKLE SPRAIN

Enter 1/2" anterior to the lateral malleolus for the talofibular ligament and 1/2" below the tip of the lateral malleolus for the fibulocalcaneal ligament.

Needle: 5/8", 25 gauge

Depth: 1/2 to 5/8"

Volume: 1 to 2 ml of anesthetic; 0.5 ml of D80

Note: confirm the placement with local anesthetic first; immobilize for 3 to 4 weeks after the injection.

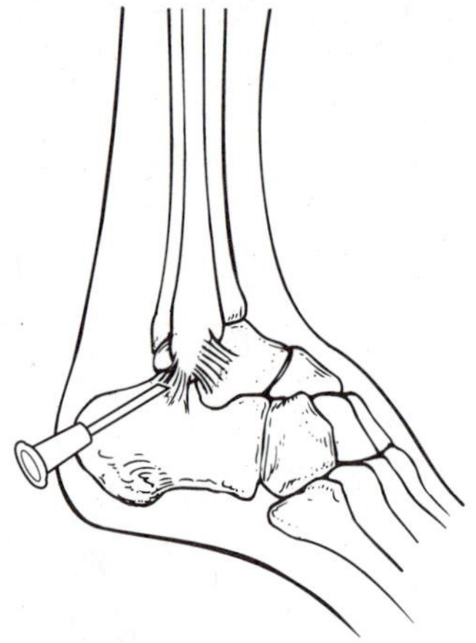

Figure 10–1. Fibulocalcaneal ligament injection.

Description An ankle sprain is a partial tear of the supporting ligaments of the ankle joint. Inversion injuries cause the fibulocalcaneal or the fibulotalar ligaments to pull away from their normal bony attachments. Sprains are classified as acute, recurrent, or chronic. Ligaments that do not heal properly and do not reattach to their bony origins can cause significant ankle joint instability, which in turn can lead to osteochondritis dissecans or osteoarthritis.

Symptoms The patient has ankle pain, ankle swelling and bruising, or instability of the ankle (in the recurrent or chronic case).

''I stepped off a high curb, higher than I thought, and came down on the side of my foot. My ankle immediately swelled, and I couldn't put any weight on it.''

''I tried to turn a corner while running, and my ankle suddenly gave out.''

''I jumped up and landed on the side of my foot. Ever since, I have had sharp pain along the outside.''

''I injured my ankle years ago, and it has been weak ever since.''

''My ankle is all swollen and black and blue on the side.''

''Four weeks ago I sprained my ankle. I had this huge black-and-blue spot that went away. My ankle still feels weak.''

''Every time I try and play B-ball my ankle gives out. I wear high-top shoes, but I still can't run or jump as well.''

Exam Each patient should be examined for irritation, inflammation, and laxity of the individual lateral ankle ligaments along with an evaluation of ankle function, swelling, and instability.

EXAM SUMMARY

1. Tenderness, swelling, or bruising anterior and inferior to the lateral malleolus
2. Pain aggravated by forced ankle inversion
3. Negative isometrics of plantarflexion and eversion
4. Full range of motion of the ankle (in the nonacute case)
5. Ankle instability (positive drawer sign or talar knock sign)

(1) Minor ankle sprains are tender anterior and inferior to the lateral malleolus. Moderate-to-severe ankle sprains have tenderness combined with swelling and bruising. The acute and severe ankle sprain may be so intensely sore that the remaining portions of the exam are not possible. (2) As the acute symptoms resolve, forced inversion of the ankle aggravates the pain. This should improve gradually as the condition resolves. (3) Isometric testing of the peroneus tendons may demonstrate pain inferior to the lateral malleolus (active tendinitis) or may demonstrate pain and tenderness at the insertion on the fifth metatarsal (avulsion fracture). (4) The range of motion of the ankle should be normal once the acute symptoms have resolved. (5) Long-standing recurrent or chronic cases may show instability of the ankle. An anterior or posterior drawer sign may be present. Rocking the ankle back and forth passively may produce a knocking, the talar knock sign. The latter usually indicates a separation of the interosseous membrane between the tibia and the fibula. Lastly, long-standing ankle instability may lead to signs of limited range of motion, crepitation, and pain at the extremes of motion (i.e., osteoarthritis of the ankle).

X-Rays   Plain films of the ankle are routinely ordered to exclude an avulsion fracture. These flecks of bone are difficult to detect and may require oblique views for confirmation. Most films are normal. Patients with persistent localized findings may benefit from magnetic resonance imaging (MRI) scanning. Osteochondritis dissecans or early arthritic changes may be seen.

Diagnosis   The diagnosis is based on the history of inversion injury coupled with the obvious physical findings. Plain x-ray films are used only to exclude avulsion fractures or frank fractures of the bones. Rarely, regional anesthetic block over the affected ligament is necessary to differentiate irritation of one periarticular structure from another.

Treatment   The goals of treatment are to allow the lateral ligaments of the ankle to reattach to their bony insertions, to strengthen the tendons that cross the ankle, and to prevent recurrent ankle sprains.

Step 1: Limit weightbearing.

Immobilize with an Ace wrap and crutches, overlap-taping, an air cast, a short-leg walking cast, or an Unna boot (pp. 162 to 163).

(Note that owing to the high rate of recurrence of poorly healing ligament injuries, erring on the side of more rigid immobilization is suggested!)

Apply ice and elevate the ankle.

Step 2 (1 to 3 weeks): Do gentle stretch exercises.

Do isometric toning.

Wear a Velcro ankle brace (p. 182) or high-top tennis shoes.

Limit some activities, especially stop-and-go sports, basketball, running, and impact aerobics.

Educate the patient, "Healing is measured in months rather than weeks. Be patient."

Step 3 (6 to 8 weeks): Give a local injection with D80 coupled with a short-leg walking cast.

Repeat the injection in 4 to 6 weeks if symptoms have not been reduced by 50%.

Re-emphasize the need to perform daily stretch and toning exercises.

Physical Therapy   Physical therapy plays an essential role in the active treatment and rehabilitation of an ankle sprain.

PHYSICAL THERAPY SUMMARY

1. Ice and elevation for acute pain and swelling
2. Heating and ankle stretching for postimmobilization rehabilitation
3. Isometric toning exercises to strengthen the ankle

ACUTELY   Ice and elevation are used in the first few days to effectively reduce the acute pain and swelling. Fifteen- to 20-minute treatments several times a day will reduce tissue distortion from bleeding and swelling.

RECOVERY/REHABILITATION   After the acute pain and swelling have subsided, exercises are performed to restore normal range of motion and to strengthen the ankle joint. *Stretch exercises* of the ankle joint are performed after fixed immobilization, especially with casting. Dorsiflexion and plantarflexion stretching are performed initially followed by gentle inversion and eversion. The ankle is heated prior to exercise. Sets of 20 passive stretches in each direction are performed daily. These stretches are necessary prior to resuming normal activities. *Isometric exercises* are used to strengthen and stabilize the ankle joint in order to prevent recurrent sprains (p. 164). Toning of the supporting tendons is necessary to overcome the weakness of a torn or severely separated ankle ligament.

Injection Technique   Immobilization is the treatment of choice. Local injection is not commonly performed and is reserved for persistently painful and swollen ankles.

Position: The patient is placed in the supine position with the ankle in a neutral position.

Technique: The tip of the lateral malleolus is identified. A 25-gauge needle is inserted either anterior to or just below the tip (depending on the injured ligament) and advanced to the bone. The needle is withdrawn 4 mm so that the medication is placed just on top of the ligament. After a local anesthetic block, the ankle is re-examined to confirm the diagnosis and the exact placement of the Xylocaine. If the stretch signs are no longer painful and local tenderness has been relieved, then ½ ml of D80 is injected in the same exact area.

Restrictions: The patient is placed in a short-leg walker or an air cast for the next 3 to 4 weeks. With improvement the cast is removed, gentle stretch exercises are performed for the next several days and toning exercises are begun in 5 to 7 days. A Velcro ankle brace is suggested for vigorous activities.

Prognosis   Always carefully examine and treat ankle sprains. Improper immobilization with nonanatomic healing can lead to weak ankles or to recurrent-chronic ankle sprains. It is better to treat aggressively with rigid immobilization than to undertreat with inadequate protection. Surgery is reserved for unstable joints with positive

---

ACHILLES TENDINITIS

Enter at the outer edge of the tendon, approximately 1" above the calcaneus.

Needle: 1 1/2 ", 22 gauge

Depth: superficial — 3/8 to 1/2"

Volume: 2 to 3 ml of anesthetic; 0.5 ml of D80 on either side of the tendon

Note: do not enter the tendon; inject along the sides with minimal pressure.

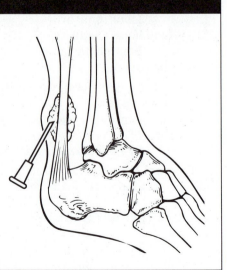

Figure 10–2.   Achilles tendon injection.

drawer signs, a positive talar knock sign, or inversion instability. Only 5 to 10% would qualify for surgical intervention.

Description   Achilles tendinitis is an inflammation of the musculotendinous junction of the Achilles tendon. Repetitive irritation and persistent inflammation lead to microtearing. Runners, patients with short Achilles tendons, and patients with Reiter's disease are at particular risk. Dramatic changes in the level of activity, improper warm-up prior to activity, and inadequate stretching of the tendon predispose to irritation. Untreated smoldering tendinitis may be complicated by acute rupture (up to 10% of cases) or chronic tendinitis.

Symptoms   The patient has ankle pain and painful walking, standing, or weight-bearing sports activities.

"I have to stop running after 2 miles because the back of my ankle begins to ache."

"I get sharp pain through my ankle and up the back of my leg whenever I jump."

"My shoes feel like they're rubbing against the bone."

"I've had to shorten my jogging stride because my cords hurt."

"My Achilles tendon is larger on the right side."

"If I try to do my leg stretches, I get a sharp pain up the back of my leg."

"I was playing basketball when I got this sudden shock of pain right behind my ankle. I looked back to see who might have kicked me, but no one was there. Every step I take now hurts behind my ankle."

Exam   Each patient should be examined for Achilles tendon irritation, paratendinous thickening, and rupture.

EXAM SUMMARY

---

1. Tenderness and "cobblestone" thickening 1½" above the calcaneus
2. Pain aggravated by resisting plantarflexion isometrically
3. Pain aggravated by passive stretching in dorsiflexion
4. The range of motion of the ankle is otherwise normal
5. The strength and tendon integrity are intact

---

(1) The Achilles tendon is enlarged at the musculotendinous juncture. The thickening is 1 to 1½" above the calcaneal insertion, fusiform in shape, and cobblestone-like to the touch. The entire area is sensitive to pressure, especially from side compression. (2) The pain is aggravated by resisting active plantarflexion isometrically and (3) by passive stretching in dorsiflexion. (4) The range of motion of the ankle is preserved, although pain may limit the ability to measure dorsiflexion accurately. (5) Palpation of the length of the tendon is free of defects. The strength of the calf muscles is preserved.

X-Rays   Plain films of the ankle and lower extremity bony structures are normal. Calcification does not occur at the musculoskeletal junction; however, incidental calcification of the calcaneal insertion of the tendon occurs frequently but should not be misdiagnosed as a sign of tendinitis. MRI scanning can provide significant additional information, especially on persistent cases and on cases considered for surgery. Paratendinous swelling, degenerative change, partial- and full-thickness tears can be demonstrated.

Diagnosis   The diagnosis is based on the examination of tenderness and thickening of the tendon, aggravated by passive stretching and isometric tension. MRI scanning is very useful in separating the uncomplicated case from those associated with partial- or full-thickness tendon rupture. Alternatively, a regional anesthetic block followed by careful retesting may disclose subtle weakness or difficult-to-feel tendon separations.

Treatment   The goals of treatment are to reduce the peritendinous swelling and thickening, to allow the microtears of the tendon to heal, to prevent frank rupture of the tendon, and to gradually stretch out the muscle and tendon to prevent a recurrence. Note that patients present with varying degrees of tendon irritation, from minor stiffness to frank tendon rupture. Treatment must be individualized.

Step 1: Rest and reduce weightbearing.

> Suggest crutches for 7 to 10 days if symptoms are hyperacute.
> Apply ice.
> Shorten the stride when walking.
> Use padded heel cups or a heel lift (p. 185).
> Use "New Skin," moleskin, or double socks to reduce friction (p. 182).
> Wear "V-notched" tennis shoes.

Step 2 (3 to 6 weeks): A NSAID (e.g., ibuprofen [Advil, Motrin]) at full dosage for 3 to 4 weeks.

> Use a Velcro ankle brace or air cast (pp. 182 to 183).

Step 3 (6 to 8 weeks): Give a local injection of D80 coupled with an air cast or short-leg walking cast ("in equinous").

Step 4 (10 to 12 weeks): Do stretch exercises daily followed by toning exercises (pp. 163 to 164).

> Wear high-top tennis shoes.
> Increase activities very gradually (10% increases in time or distance each week; alternate running days with weight training, etc.).
> Continue to reduce friction over the back of the heel.
> Limit high-impact sports, jumping, and long-distance running or consider an orthopedic consultation if swelling and pain are persistent.

Physical Therapy   Physical therapy plays an important role in the treatment and rehabilitation of Achilles tendinitis.

PHYSICAL THERAPY SUMMARY

> 1. Ice
> 2. Phonophoresis with hydrocortisone gel
> 3. Passive stretching
> 4. Active stretching
> 5. Isometric toning

ACUTELY   Ice and phonophoresis are used in the first few weeks to reduce the acute pain and welling. *Ice* or phonophoresis applied to the musculotendinous junction provides short-term relief of pain and swelling. *Gentle passive stretching* is always recommended during the later phases of active treatment. A foreshortened, inflexible tendon is susceptible to continued irritation. Stretching applied with hand pressure and very gentle wall stretches should be performed daily (p. 163). Mild discomfort in the calf is normal, but acute or sharp pain in the tendon area must be avoided. These are performed after heating.

RECOVERY/REHABILITATION   Complete healing requires continued daily stretching, and prevention requires stretching and toning of the tendon. *Passive stretching* exercises are continued in the recovery period. Vigorous stretching exercises to achieve 30 degrees of dorsiflexion are started 3 to 4 weeks after the acute symptoms have resolved. Once full dorsiflexion has been obtained, *isometric toning exercises* are begun. These exercises should be performed daily using a TheraBand, large rubber bands, or a bungy cord. Sets of 20 are performed with the ankle kept in neutral position. As strength and tone increase, weightbearing active toning exercises can be performed (p. 163). With increasing strength, full weightbearing activities can be resumed.

Injection Technique Rest, restriction of activities, and immobilization are the mainstays of treatment. The role of local injection is still controversial. Local corticosteroid injection can effectively reduce the chronic peritendinous inflammation and thickening; however, the need to arrest the ongoing chronic inflammatory reaction must be balanced against the potential risk of postinjection tendon rupture. Thus, any local injection must be combined with rigid immobilization.

Position: The patient is placed prone on the exam table with the foot hanging over the end of the exam table. The ankle is kept in neutral position.

Technique: The area of maximum tendon thickening is identified, typically 1 to 1½″ above the calcaneus. Local anesthesia is placed on either side of the tendon, adjacent to and slightly below the thickening. If local tenderness is significantly relieved and the strength of dorsiflexion is preserved, then ½ ml of D80 is injected on either side of the tendon, peritendinously!

Restrictions: A short-leg walking cast in the equinus position is used for the next 3 weeks. After cast removal, the tendon is gradually stretched and toned for several weeks (p. 163). Activities are gradually resumed.

Prognosis Achilles tendinitis can be dishearteningly persistent or recurrent, probably owing to the degree of underlying microtearing of the tendon and persistent inflammation. Stepped care from simple rest and reduction in running schedule and stretch exercise is always a good starting point; however, simple conservative care should not be prolonged indefinitely. Chronic inflammation around and through the tendon probably contributes in a major way to spontaneous tendon ruptures. Persistent inflammation must be treated in a timely fashion. Local injection should be considered at 2 to 3 months or earlier if tendon thickening is great and later if it is minimal. All spontaneous tendon ruptures and most cases of persistent tendinitis should be seen by the orthopedic surgeon. Primary tendon repair can be combined with surgical stripping of the peritendinous tissue or sharp dissection of the mucinoid degeneration.

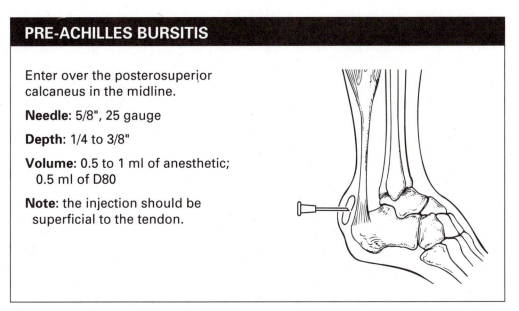

PRE-ACHILLES BURSITIS

Enter over the posterosuperior calcaneus in the midline.

Needle: 5/8″, 25 gauge

Depth: 1/4 to 3/8″

Volume: 0.5 to 1 ml of anesthetic; 0.5 ml of D80

Note: the injection should be superficial to the tendon.

Figure 10–3. Pre-Achilles bursa injection.

Description   Pre-Achilles bursitis is an inflammation of the bursal sac, located between the calcaneal insertion of the Achilles tendon and the overlying skin. Its function is to reduce the friction between the skin and the tendon. Although frequently misdiagnosed as Achilles tendinitis, it is distinctly different. Pre-Achilles bursitis is rarely disabling and does not lead to tendon rupture.

Symptoms   The patient has pain and localized swelling behind the heel.

"I can't find a comfortable pair of shoes. I can't stand any pressure over the back of my heel."

"There's a lump over the back of my heel."

"My doctor tells me that I have a calcium deposit over the back of my heel."

"The back of my heel hurts."

Exam   Each patient should be examined for local bursal tenderness and swelling.

EXAM SUMMARY

---

1. Local tenderness and swelling just over the posterior calcaneus
2. Minimal pain with passive stretching in dorsiflexion
3. Resisted plantarflexion is painless
4. Normal range of motion of the ankle

---

(1) Local tenderness and swelling are present directly over the posterior calcaneus. The quarter-sized area of inflammation is 1" superior to the heel pad, directly in the midline. (2) Passive stretching of the Achilles tendon in dorsiflexion and (3) active resisted plantarflexion are minimally painful. This is in contrast to the exam of acute Achilles tendinitis! The range of motion of the ankle is normal.

X-Rays   Plain films of the ankle are often ordered but are not necessary for the diagnosis. The lateral view of the ankle often shows calcification either arising from the superior process of the calcaneus or as a discrete calcification in the bursa. Calcification does not necessarily influence the clinical decision-making, although deposits measuring 1 cm in length may present a pressure effect in and of themselves.

Diagnosis   The diagnosis is based on the swelling and tenderness in the characteristic location over the superior calcaneus. A regional anesthetic block is rarely necessary to distinguish superficial involvement of the bursa from the underlying bony lesion.

Treatment   The goals of treatment are to reduce the friction over the heel, to reduce the inflammation in the bursa, and to prevent a recurrence of Achilles stretching.

Step 1: Reduce heel friction with padded heel cups, moleskin, double socks, or "New Skin" (p. 182).
> Use a large felt ring (p. 187).
> Use fleece heel pads while lying in bed.
> Avoid shoes with rigid backs.
> Consider "V-notched" tennis shoes.
> Shorten the walking or running stride.
> Do Achilles stretch exercises (p. 163).

Step 2 (3 to 6 weeks): Give a local injection with D80.
> Re-emphasize step 1.

Step 3 (8 to 10 weeks): Repeat the injection in 4 to 6 weeks if symptoms are not relieved by at least 50% or combine the injection with a walking cast.

Physical Therapy   Physical therapy plays an adjunctive role to immobilization and local injection in the treatment of pre-Achilles bursitis. Ice is a very effective analgesic, since the bursa is located in the superficial tissues, ⅜″ below the skin surface. Stretching exercises of the Achilles tendon are generally helpful (p. 163). Immobilization and local injection are indicated for persistent cases.

Injection Technique   Measures to reduce friction are the preferred initial steps of treatment. Local injection is very useful but must often be combined with immobilization for optimal results.

Position: The patient is placed prone with the foot over the edge of the table. The ankle is kept in neutral position.

Technique: The center of the bursa is identified, typically in the midline over the posterosuperior angle of the calcaneus. The skin is puckered into the midline to facilitate entry of the needle. The needle is advanced down to the firm tissue resistance of the tendon (either felt as a harder tissue to advance through or as firmer tissue to inject into). The anesthetic is injected over a dime-sized area. The patient is re-examined. If significant pain relief has occurred, a ½ ml of D80 is injected. Firm pressure may be needed when injecting into this tense tissue layer.

Restrictions: Activities are kept to a minimum for the first few days. Measures to control friction and pressure over the area must be reinforced. Persistent cases should be immobilized postinjection with a short-leg walking cast or air cast (p. 183).

Prognosis   This lower extremity pressure-sensitive bursa may be difficult to heal. Retreatment is not unusual. Emphasis has to be placed on protection and prevention. Bursectomy is rarely suggested.

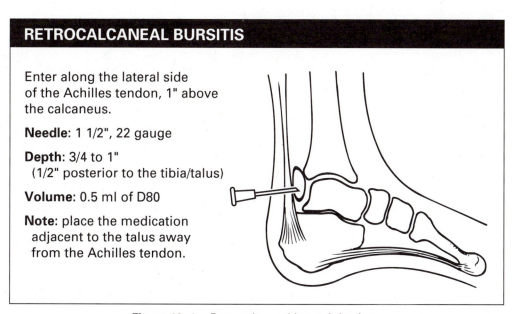

RETROCALCANEAL BURSITIS

Enter along the lateral side of the Achilles tendon, 1" above the calcaneus.

Needle: 1 1/2", 22 gauge

Depth: 3/4 to 1"
(1/2" posterior to the tibia/talus)

Volume: 0.5 ml of D80

Note: place the medication adjacent to the talus away from the Achilles tendon.

Figure 10–4.   Retrocalcaneal bursa injection.

Description   Retrocalcaneal bursitis is an inflammation of the bursal sac located between the Achilles tendon and the posterior aspect of the ankle. It lubricates the tendon and the talus bone when the foot is in extreme plantarflexion.

Symptoms   The patient has ankle pain (behind the ankle) and painful walking.

"The back of my ankle hurts whenever I go upstairs too fast."

"My knee has been swollen, and I've been limping. Now I have a pain in the back of my ankle."

"I can't see any swelling. My ankle still moves okay, but I'm having this pain behind my ankle every time I walk."

Exam   Each patient should be examined for local tenderness and swelling in the soft tissues behind the ankle along with an evaluation of Achilles tendon flexibility.

EXAM SUMMARY

1. Local tenderness and swelling between the Achilles tendon and the ankle
2. Pain is aggravated by passive forced plantarflexion
3. Isometric tension applied to the ankle tendons is painless
4. Range of motion of the ankle is normal

(1) Local tenderness and swelling are present in the soft tissue space between the Achilles tendon and the posterior ankle. Pressure applied to the soft tissues just posterior to the talus is painful. Severe cases may swell dramatically, filling in the space between the talus and the Achilles tendon. (2) Pain is aggravated by passively forcing the foot into severe plantarflexion, thus compressing the bursa. (3) Isometric testing of the tendons that cross the ankle do not aggravate the pain. Resisted dorsiflexion, plantarflexion, inversion, and eversion are painless. (4) The range of motion of the ankle is normal.

X-Rays   Plain films are not necessary for the diagnosis. Calcification does not occur. Ankle views may be necessary in a long distance runner to exclude a stress fracture of the calcaneus.

Diagnosis   A presumptive diagnosis is based on the characteristic local tenderness aggravated by passive plantarflexion. The diagnosis is confirmed by a regional anesthetic block placed in the bursa adjacent to the talus.

Treatment   The goals of treatment are to reduce the swelling and inflammation in the bursa and to prevent a recurrence by Achilles tendon stretch exercises.

Step 1: Restrict repetitive ankle motion (e.g., limit stairs, walk on flat surfaces, no jumping or jogging).
    Avoid high heels.
    Shorten the stride when walking.
    Use padded heel cups (p. 185).

Step 2 (3 to 6 weeks): Use of an NSAID (e.g., ibuprofen [Advil, Motrin]) has limited benefit.
    Apply a Velcro ankle brace (p. 182).

Step 3 (6 to 8 weeks): Give a local injection with K40.
    Continue the restrictions and use of the brace.
    Repeat the injection in 4 to 6 weeks if symptoms have not decreased by 50%.

Step 4 (10 to 12 weeks): Do stretch exercises for the Achilles tendon (p. 163).
    Gradually resume regular activities.

Physical Therapy   Physical therapy does not play an important role in the treatment of retrocalcaneal bursitis. Ice and elevation are always recommended for pain and swelling along with the recommendations for the general care of the ankle (pp. 162 to 164). No other treatments are specific for this isolated bursitis.

Injection Technique   Local injection is the treatment of choice if symptoms fail to respond to rest and restricted use.

Position: The patient is placed in the prone position with the foot hanging over the end of the exam table. The ankle is kept in neutral position.

Technique: The needle is inserted halfway between the Achilles tendon and the lateral portion of the talus, approximately 1″ above the calcaneus. The needle is advanced down to the middle of the talus. The anesthetic is injected in the midline just posterior to the talus. If the local tenderness and pain with forced plantar flexion are relieved, ½ ml of K40 is injected.

Restrictions: Restrict repetitious ankle motion for 3 days, and limit the use for the next 30 days. Continue to wear the ankle brace for 30 days.

Prognosis   Local injection is very effective. Achilles stretching and strengthening will decrease the likelihood of a recurrence. A bursectomy is not performed.

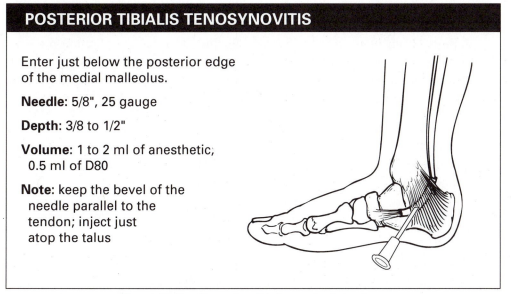

POSTERIOR TIBIALIS TENOSYNOVITIS

Enter just below the posterior edge of the medial malleolus.

Needle: 5/8″, 25 gauge

Depth: 3/8 to 1/2″

Volume: 1 to 2 ml of anesthetic; 0.5 ml of D80

Note: keep the bevel of the needle parallel to the tendon; inject just atop the talus

Figure 10–5.   Posterior tibialis tendon injection.

Description   Posterior tibialis tenosynovitis is an inflammation of the tendon as it curves around the medial malleolus. It lies in a tenosynovial sheath that lubricates it against the underside of the bone. Pronated ankles, flat feet, ankle arthritis, and excessive body weight are predisposing factors. In cases of severe pronation, this tenosynovitis may be accompanied by the entrapment of the posterior tibial nerve, tarsal tunnel syndrome.

Symptoms   The patient has pain and swelling on the inner aspect of the ankle and painful walking.

"I have this sharp pain around the inside of my ankle whenever I step."

"There's swelling around the back of my ankle (pointing to the inner aspect of the ankle)."

"Tight shoes have rubbed the inside of my ankle raw . . . The skin looks normal though."

Exam   Each patient should be examined for inflammation and swelling of the tendon sheath along with an assessment of ankle range of motion and alignment.

EXAM SUMMARY

> **1.** Local tenderness and swelling just inferior and posterior to the medial malleolus
> **2.** Pain aggravated by resisting ankle inversion and plantarflexion isometrically.
> **3.** Pain may be aggravated by passive stretching in eversion
> **4.** Normal range of motion of the ankle
> **5.** Pronated ankles, pes planus, or pes cavus?

(1) Local tenderness and swelling are located in a crescent-shaped area inferior and posterior to the medial malleolus. The swelling may be so dramatic as to fill in the dimpling below the inferior tip of the malleolus. (2) The pain is consistently aggravated by resisting the action of the tendon isometrically. Inversion is usually more painful than resisting plantarflexion. (3) The pain may be aggravated by forced eversion of the ankle, passively performed. (4) The range of motion of the ankle is normal in an uncomplicated case. (5) Pes planus, pes cavus, or ankle pronation may be present.

X-Rays   Plain films are not necessary for the diagnosis. Calcification does not occur. Ankle views are normal unless there is a concomitant arthritic process.

Diagnosis   A presumptive diagnosis is based on the history of medial ankle pain, an exam showing local tenderness and swelling in the characteristic crescent-shaped area inferior and posterior to the medial malleolus, and pain aggravated by isometric tension of the tendon. A regional anesthetic block confirms the diagnosis and will differentiate this pain from the pain arising from the ankle joint or tarsal tunnel.

Treatment   The goals of treatment are to reduce the inflammation in the tendon sheath and to correct any underlying abnormalities of ankle alignment.

Step 1: Evaluate and correct ankle pronation (high-top shoes, arch supports, or a medial wedge), pes planus (arch supports), or metatarsalgia (padded insoles).
Limit standing and walking.
Apply ice.
Use a Velcro pull-on ankle brace (p. 182).
Use an NSAID (e.g., ibuprofen [Advil, Motrin]) for 4 weeks.

Step 2 (6 to 8 weeks): Give a local injection with D80, combined with a short-leg walking cast (p. 183).
Give another injection with D80 if symptoms have not improved by 50%.
Combine the second injection with a cast or a tight-fitting Velcro ankle brace.

Step 3 (8 to 10 weeks): Gently stretch the ankle in all four directions.
Consider custom-made plaster-molded rigid orthotics.

Physical Therapy   Physical therapy is important in the rehabilitation of posterior tibialis tenosynovitis in the postcasting recovery period. Gradual stretching exercise of the ankle (emphasizing dorsiflexion and eversion) are performed daily (p. 163). These exercises are performed after heating the ankle in sets of 20. They are begun immediately after casting or approximately 4 weeks after local injection.

Injection Technique   Successful treatment of this tendon inflammation must combine abnormal ankle alignment correction with local injection. To guard against the possibility of postinjection tendon rupture (which is rare), casting is used concurrently.

Position: The patient is placed in the supine position with the leg fully extended and the lower leg rotated externally.

Technique: The tip of the medial malleolus is identified. The needle enters just behind the posterior edge of it and is advanced down to the medial talus. The bevel of the needle is kept parallel to the course of the tendon fibers. Once the bone is touched, the needle is withdrawn 1 to 2 mm, and the medication is injected. Minimal pressure is necessary if the needle is in the tenosynovial sheath. If the local tenderness and isometric pain with resisted ankle inversion are dramatically improved, then ½ ml of D80 is injected.

Restrictions: Following injection, a short-leg walking cast is used for 3 weeks. Stretch and toning exercises of the tendon are begun in the fourth week.

Prognosis   An injection combined with immobilization is usually successful. Recurrent tenosynovitis often occurs in the setting of difficult-to-manage ankle instability, ankle deformity, obesity, or old trauma. Surgery is usually reserved for tendon rupture (which is rare).

PLANTAR FASCIITIS

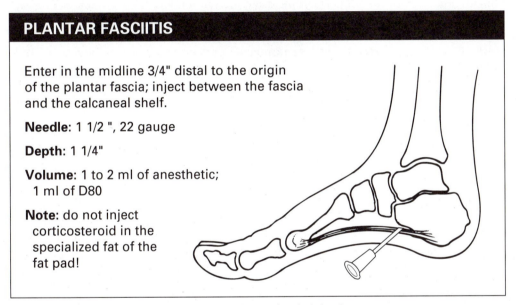

Enter in the midline 3/4" distal to the origin of the plantar fascia; inject between the fascia and the calcaneal shelf.

Needle: 1 1/2 ", 22 gauge

Depth: 1 1/4"

Volume: 1 to 2 ml of anesthetic; 1 ml of D80

Note: do not inject corticosteroid in the specialized fat of the fat pad!

Figure 10–6.   Plantar fascia injection.

Description   Plantar fasciitis is an inflammation of the origin of the longitudinal ligament that forms the arch of the foot. Flat feet (pes planus), high arches (pes cavus), turned-in ankles (ankle pronation), and short Achilles tendons predispose to this condition. Obesity, working on concrete, poorly fitted shoes, and prolonged daily standing aggravate the condition. A few cases are purely inflammatory in nature and are associated with Reiter's syndrome.

Symptoms   The patient has heel pain aggravated by walking and standing.

"Whenever I put pressure down on my heel, I get a severe, sharp pain under my heel."

"The pressure over my heel is so bad that I have started to walk on my tiptoes."

"My flat feet never bothered me until I took this job where I have to walk or stand on concrete all day long."

"I can't wear these kinds of shoes (flats) because my heel will really start to hurt."

"It's like the bottom of my heel is bruised."

"I can't wear high heels any more because my heel hurts."

"I can't do my Jazzercise any more because of my heel."

Exam   Each patient should be examined for local irritation and inflammation of the fascia along with an evaluation of ankle alignment, Achilles tendon flexibility, and the configuration of the arch of the foot.

EXAM SUMMARY

1. Local tenderness at the calcaneal origin of the plantar fascia
2. Pain with calcaneal compression
3. Achilles tendon inflexibility
4. Associated ankle pronation, pes planus, and pes cavus
5. Anesthetic block at the origin

(1) Local tenderness is present in the midline of the foot at the origin of the longitudinal arch of the foot. The dime-sized area of tenderness is located 1¼ to 1½" from the posterior heel. Firm pressure may be needed! (2) Medial to lateral compression of the calcaneus may be mildly painful but rarely more painful than the local tenderness! A stress fracture of the calcaneus is suggested if calcaneal compression is more painful than the local tenderness at the plantar fascial origin. (3) Achilles tendon flexibility may be limited. The tendon often shortens as a result of a shortened stride or favoring the foot. Normally, the ankle should dorsiflex to 25 to 30 degrees. (4) Ankle pronation, pes planus, or pes cavus may be associated findings. It is mandatory to examine the arch and the ankle alignment in the standing position!

X-Rays   Plain films of the ankle are not necessary to make the diagnosis. They are indicated in long distance runners to exclude a stress fracture of the calcaneus, in patients with injuries to exclude a routine fracture, and in patients with chronic symptoms to exclude a large (> 1 cm) heel spur that may require surgical excision. Small calcaneal calcifications at the origin of the fascia are exceedingly common; they are a reflection of the inflammatory process. Small heel spurs, protected by the shelf of the calcaneus, are not an indication for surgery in and of themselves!

Diagnosis   The diagnosis is based on the history of plantar heel pain and on the characteristic local tenderness. A regional anesthetic block at the origin can be used to differentiate the heel pad syndrome, calcaneal stress fracture, and plantar fasciitis.

Treatment   The goals of treatment are to reduce the inflammation in the longitudinal arch and to improve the mechanics of heel and ankle motion.

Step 1: Cushion the heel with heel cups, foam to stand on at work, padded insoles, or double socks (p. 185).

Limit standing and walking.
Wear padded arch supports (e.g., Spenco, Sorbothane) (pp. 185 to 186).
Wear comfortable, well-supporting shoes.
Apply ice.
Do Achilles tendon stretch exercises (p. 163).
Massage over the heel with a rubber ball.

Step 2 (3 to 4 weeks): An NSAID (e.g., ibuprofen [Advil, Motrin]) may help.
Re-emphasize the use of padding.

Step 3 (6 to 8 weeks): X-ray the heel.

Give a local injection with D80.
Give a repeat injection in 4 to 6 weeks if symptoms have not decreased by 50%.
Consider a short-leg walking cast with the repeat injection (p. 183).

Step 4 (3 to 4 months): Consider a referral to a podiatrist for custom-made orthotics (p. 186) or surgical débridement.

Physical Therapy Physical therapy plays a significant role in the active treatment of plantar fasciitis and in its prevention.

PHYSICAL THERAPY SUMMARY

> **1.** Ice
> **2.** Heat and massage to the heel
> **3.** Achilles tendon stretching

ACUTELY Ice, massage, and padding are used in the first several weeks to reduce pain and swelling. *Ice* placed over the center of the heel provides effective analgesia and may help to reduce swelling. Cold must be applied for 10 to 15 minutes in order to penetrate ¾ to 1″ down to the origin of the fascia. For other patients, *heating and massage* provides more effective analgesia and may help to disperse swelling. This can be accomplished with a tennis ball rolled under the heel or with a vibrating foot massage unit.

RECOVERY/REHABILITATION After the acute symptoms have significantly decreased, stretching exercises are begun. The most important treatment for plantar fasciitis is *Achilles stretching exercises* (p. 163). Increasing Achilles tendon flexibility lessens the tension over the plantar fascia. The fascia, calcaneus, and Achilles tendon must share the workload of ankle motion. Stiffness in one area will increase the tension and stress in other areas. Passive and active stretching exercises are performed daily. When combined with padded insoles, arch supports, and well-supported shoes, plantar fasciitis is less likely to recur.

Injection Technique The emphasis in early treatment is on mechanical rest and padding. If inflammation persists, a local injection is usually effective. Difficult cases may require two injections and rigid immobilization.

Position: The patient is placed in the prone position with the foot hanging just off the edge of the exam table.

Technique: The origin of the plantar fascia is identified approximately 1 to 1½″ from the back of the heel. The needle enters ¾″ distal to the origin and is advanced at a 45-degree angle down to the firm resistance of the fascia (~ 1″ in depth at this angle of entry!). A ½ ml of anesthetic is placed at the fascia, and then the needle is advanced through it and down to the shelf of the calcaneus. Often a giving way will be felt as the 22-gauge needle penetrates through the fascia. A small amount of anesthetic is injected between the fascia and the bone (usually only ½ ml is used because the space is limited). If the local tenderness is significantly relieved, 1 ml of D80 is injected slowly.

Restrictions: Weightbearing is limited for 3 days. Prolonged standing, long walking, and running are limited for 30 days. Persistent cases can be immobilized for 3 to 4 weeks in a walking cast.

Prognosis Local injection alone is successful in approximately 60% of cases. When one or two injections are combined with a cast for 3 to 4 weeks, most patients resolve the condition. Persistent or recurrent fasciitis is seen most often in patients with obesity, with abnormal arch and ankle conditions, or with jobs demanding prolonged standing or walking on concrete surfaces. Surgical débridement of the devitalized tissue or the accompanying bone spur (if the spur is greater than 1 cm) is occasionally indicated.

BUNIONS

Enter over the metatarsophalangeal joint medially at the distal metatarsal head.

Needle: 5/8", 25 gauge

Depth: 3/8 to 5/8" (flush against the bone)

Volume: 0.5 ml of anesthetic; 0.25 ml of D80

Note: the injection is made under the synovial lining adjacent to the bone, not in the joint itself!

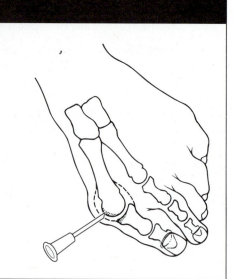

Figure 10–7. Bunion injection.

Description   A bunion is a descriptive term used to define the prominence and abnormal angle of the first metatarsophalangeal (MTP) joint, resulting from osteoarthritis. Narrow toe-box shoes, the asymmetric loss of articular cartilage, and the gradual subluxation of the extensor tendons cause the typical valgus deformity. The condition develops over many years and commonly affects family members. Continued pressure over the medial joint line can cause acute arthritic flares and can produce an acute adventitial bursitis.

Symptoms   The patient complains of the abnormal-looking toes, problems with "shoe wear" and "toe pain" in the great toe.

"I can't get a pair of shoes to fit comfortably now."

"I get this sharp pain in my big toe whenever I walk too far."

"My toe looks funny."

"Are these bunions? My grandmother had ugly toes too."

"My big toe aches all the time, especially when I bend it."

"My big toe doesn't bend very much any more."

Exam   Each patient should be examined for arthritic change, valgus angulation, and local inflammation involving the first MTP joint.

EXAM SUMMARY

1. Hallux valgus deformity
2. MTP joint enlargement
3. Crepitation on passive movement of the joint
4. Pain at the extremes of passive plantarflexion and dorsiflexion of the toe
5. Limited range of motion

(1) The hallux valgus deformity is characterized by a prominent medial metatarsal head, an abnormal lateral angulation of the proximal phalanges, or overlapping of the first and second toes. (2) Subluxation of the MTP joint, bony osteophyte formation, or joint swelling contribute to the enlargement of the MTP joint. (3) Passive movement of the joint may cause crepitation. (4) Pain may be present at the extremes of plantar-flexion and dorsiflexion, passively performed. (5) The range of motion of the joint may be limited.

X-Rays   X-rays of the foot are recommended. Plain films will confirm the diagnosis, precisely measure the valgus angle, and assess the severity of osteoarthritis. Progressive arthritic changes include asymmetric narrowing of the articular cartilage, bony osteophyte formation, subchondral bony sclerosis, and subchondral cyst formation. X-rays are always a prerequisite to surgical consultation.

Diagnosis   Advanced cases are easily diagnosed by simple inspection and exam. Moderate cases may require plain films of the foot for confirmation. A regional anesthetic block is necessary occasionally, to differentiate symptoms arising at the MTP joint from symptoms arising from the adventitious bursa or from Morton neuroma.

Treatment   The goals of treatment are to reduce the pain and swelling within the MTP joint, to protect against further arthritic deterioration, and to retard the development of the valgus deformity.

Step 1: Educate the patient, "This is arthritis of the big toe."
> Wide toe-box shoes.
> Place a thick felt ring over the medial joint (p. 187).
> Place a cotton or rubber spacer between the first and second toes (p. 188).
> Use bunion shields (p. 186).
> Apply ice.

Step 2 (4 to 6 weeks): An NSAID (e.g., ibuprofen [Advil, Motrin]) may provide relief or give a local injection with D80.
> Give a repeat injection in 4 to 6 weeks if symptoms are not improved by 50%.

Step 3 (8 to 10 weeks): Consider a referral to an orthopedist or podiatrist if symptoms are persistent or if the deformity is great.

Physical Therapy   Physical therapy does not play a significant role in the treatment of bunions. Ice and elevation are always recommended for acute arthritic flares. Stretching exercises of the extensor and flexor tendons are important early in the condition before subluxation and deformity become fixed.

Injection Technique   Local injection can provide temporary relief for this progressive arthritic condition.

Position: The patient is placed in the supine position with the leg kept straight.

Technique: A medial approach to the joint is safest and easiest to perform. The head of the first metatarsal and the MTP joint line are palpated. A 25-gauge needle is inserted over the metatarsal perpendicular to the skin and is advanced down to the bone. The injection is placed flush with the bone, under the synovial membrane (gentle pressure is required). If the patient's local tenderness and pain with MTP motion are significantly improved, ¼ ml of D80 is injected through the same needle.

Restrictions: Walking and standing are limited for the first 3 days and are gradually increased over the next 3 to 4 weeks. Use of padding, wide toe-box shoes, and the felt ring is continued.

Prognosis   The underlying arthritis and deformity gradually worsen over the years. Once this wear-and-tear process begins, it tends to be relentlessly progressive.

Prevention and protection cannot be overemphasized. All treatments, including surgery, are palliative.

When deformity ("hallux valgus") is dramatic, surgery can be considered. Several surgical procedures are available, providing cosmetic relief. Realignment of the MTP joint can be combined with resection of the MTP joint (proximal osteotomy, the McBride procedure, and several others). The patient should be advised that no one procedure is better than another and that the toe may lack full range of motion postoperatively. The patient must be willing to risk trading a painful deformity for a functionally stiff joint.

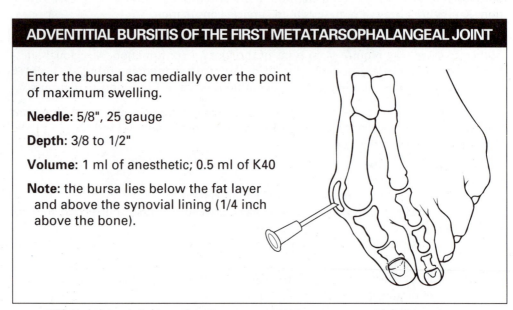

ADVENTITIAL BURSITIS OF THE FIRST METATARSOPHALANGEAL JOINT

Enter the bursal sac medially over the point of maximum swelling.

Needle: 5/8", 25 gauge

Depth: 3/8 to 1/2"

Volume: 1 ml of anesthetic; 0.5 ml of K40

Note: the bursa lies below the fat layer and above the synovial lining (1/4 inch above the bone).

Figure 10–8.   Injection of the bursa over the first metatarsophalangeal joint.

Description   A bursal sac develops over the medial aspect of the first MTP joint as a result of pressure of the underlying bony prominence. The constant pressure and friction of tight shoes causes the bursal sac to become acutely inflamed. The swelling and redness develop only along the medial aspect of the joint, as opposed to the entire MTP joint with gout.

Symptoms   The patient has toe pain, swelling, and redness, but only over the inner aspect of the toe.

"My big toe is swollen."

"I can't wear my shoes any more. My big toe rubs on the inner side of the shoe."

"I have had to switch to sandals because my walking shoes rub too much on my big toe."

"I think I have gout!"

"I've always had bunions, but now my toe has really begun to swell."

Exam   Each patient should be examined for acute inflammatory change along the medial aspect of the first MTP joint along with an evaluation of the arthritic change and loss of range of motion of the first MTP joint.

EXAM SUMMARY

> **1.** Inflammation over the medial aspect of the MTP
> **2.** Valgus deformity and arthritic change of the MTP
> **3.** Achy pain when moving the joint
> **4.** Isometrically resisted great toe flexion and extension are painless (no signs of tendinitis!)

(1) Acute inflammation is present over the medial aspect of the first MTP joint. Swelling, redness, and warmth are present over a nickel-sized area. The inflammation rarely extends beyond the bursal sac. (2) Hallux valgus is present. The MTP joint has the typical bony enlargement and acute angle. (3) The range of motion of the joint is limited due to the underlying arthritic change. Mild pain is experienced at the extremes of motion. (4) Isometrically resisted toe flexion and extension are painless. The extensor and flexor tendons of the foot are not involved.

X-Rays X-rays of the foot are recommended. The underlying arthritic change predominates. Bony spurs, joint space narrowing, and valgus deformity are usually obvious and advanced. Soft tissue swelling is greatest on the anteroposterior projection. Calcification does not occur.

Diagnosis The diagnosis is based on the characteristic swelling located over the medial joint line of an advanced hallux valgus deformity. Local anesthetic block in the soft tissue will differentiate this from the acute monoarticular inflammation of gout. Occasionally, the diagnosis can be confirmed by the aspiration of a mildly inflammatory exudate with negative crystals.

Treatment The goals of treatment are to reduce the swelling and inflammation in the bursa and to prevent a recurrence by avoiding pressure and friction.

Step 1: Wear wide toe-box shoes.
> Place a felt ring over the medial aspect of the MTP joint (p. 187).
> Use bunion shields (p. 186).
> The NSAIDs (e.g., ibuprofen [Advil, Motrin]) are ineffective.

Step 2 (3 to 4 weeks): Give a local injection of D80 or K40.
> Give a repeat injection in 4 to 6 weeks if the pain and swelling have not decreased by 50%.

Step 3 (8 to 10 weeks): Prevention is achieved with well-fitting shoes or a felt ring.

Physical Therapy Physical therapy does not play a significant role in the treatment of this condition. Ice and elevation are usually recommended. Stretching exercises of the MTP joint are indicated, just as they are for an isolated case of bunions.

Injection Technique Local injection is the treatment of choice for cases that fail conservative protection measures.

Position: The patient is placed in the prone position with the knee fully extended and the lower leg externally rotated.

Technique: The center of the bursa sac is entered medially over the MTP head. The needle is advanced down to bone and is then withdrawn ¼". (This is to ensure that the injection is placed in the tissue above the joint and not in it.) Attempts to aspirate fluid are usually unsuccessful. With the needle held in place, ½ ml of K40 is injected.

Restrictions: Walking is limited for the first 3 days. Preventative care with well-fitting shoes or a felt ring is continued for 30 days.

Prognosis Medical therapy with local injection is usually very effective. Recurrent bursitis is seen with bunions with severe angulation deformity. Surgery is usually directed to the underlying bunion. Bursectomy without surgical correction of the underlying bunion deformity is usually ineffective.

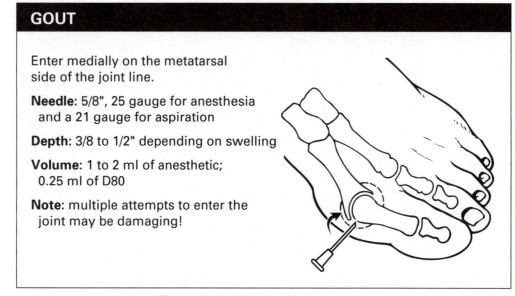

GOUT

Enter medially on the metatarsal side of the joint line.

Needle: 5/8", 25 gauge for anesthesia and a 21 gauge for aspiration

Depth: 3/8 to 1/2" depending on swelling

Volume: 1 to 2 ml of anesthetic; 0.25 ml of D80

Note: multiple attempts to enter the joint may be damaging!

Figure 10–9.   Injection for acute gout.

Description Gout is an acute monoarticular arthritis of the MTP joint of the great toe. Acute swelling, redness, and heat develop as an inflammatory response to precipitation of monosodium urate crystals in the joint fluid. There are many causes of gout. The differential diagnosis can be divided into the overproducers of uric acid (10%) and the underexcreters (90%).

Symptoms The patient has severe toe pain, swelling, and redness and an inability to walk because of the pain.

"I woke up in the night with severe, sharp pain in my big toe."

"The pain in my toe was so bad that I couldn't stand the sheets on my foot."

"My big toe is very red and swollen."

"Doc, I've got the gout in my big toe again."

"I can't put any weight down on my foot because of the severe pain in my big toe."

"There's no way I can walk. I can't bend my big toe."

"My arthritis has hurt in the past, but never like this."

Exam Each patient should be examined for the degree and extent of the inflammation affecting the great toe.

EXAM SUMMARY

1. Acute swelling, redness, and heat in the MTP joint
2. Severe tenderness at the MTP joint
3. Pain aggravated by even the slightest movement of the joint

(1) The toe is swollen, red, and hot. The inflammation may extend 1″ proximal and distal to the joint, involving the soft tissues. (2) Severe tenderness is present around the entire joint. Even the lightest touch is painful. (3) Movement of the toe in any direction is extremely painful. The patient often exhibits great anxiety at the thought of moving the toe.

X-Rays An x-ray of the foot is recommended. The x-ray of a first attack of gout is usually normal. Patients with recurrent or chronic tophaceous gout may show periarticular or intra-articular erosions that are round or oval and surrounded by a sclerotic margin.

Diagnosis A presumptive diagnosis is based on the acute monoarticular involvement of the MTP joint along with a history of gouty attacks or an elevated serum uric acid. Confirmation of the diagnosis requires demonstration of crystals on microscopic joint fluid analysis. Monosodium urate crystals are needle shaped and demonstrate negative birefringence (bright yellow) under polarized light microscopy. In addition, the joint fluid must be submitted for Gram stain and culture to exclude acute bacterial infectious arthritis! Note that gout is not restricted to the great toe. It may also cause acute dorsotenosynovitis over the extensor tendons of the foot; acute tenosynovitis of the posterior tibialis tendon of the instep; prepatellar or olecranon bursitis; or acute arthritis involving other small- and medium-sized joints.

Treatment The goal of treatment is to rapidly reduce the acute inflammation within the first MTP joint.

Step 1: Apply ice and elevate the joint.
>Eliminate alcohol, aspirin, and other drugs that increase uric acid.
>Avoid pressure from shoes.
>Any NSAID (e.g., ibuprofen [Advil, Motrin]) or colchicine or local injection of any corticosteroid derivative effectively treats the condition.
>Measure the uric acid concentration in the blood.
>Send fluid for crystals if possible.

Step 2 (within 2 to 4 weeks): Measure the 24-hour urinary uric acid excretion ("overproducer" or "underexcreter").
>Prescribe allopurinol or probenecid for long-term control of recurrent or chronic cases.
>Continue colchicine or an NSAID when beginning preventative medication at least 1 month for recurrent gout and 6 months for chronic tophaceous gout.

Step 3 (6 to 8 weeks): Recheck the uric acid.
>Adjust the dosages of allopurinol or probenecid to keep the uric acid in the normal range.

Physical Therapy Physical therapy does not play a significant role in the treatment of gout. Ice and elevation are always recommended, but definitive treatment requires medication.

Injection Technique Gout is the archetypical acute inflammatory monoarthritis. It responds dramatically to local injection! See Bunions for the specific technique (p. 117).

Prognosis The NSAIDs or colchicine should be effective within 1 to 2 days. The response to a local injection is often within hours. Either treatment will effectively control all symptoms and signs within 3 to 4 days. Long-term control of gout rests on prevention. Low-dose aspirin, alcohol, high purine–containing foods, and certain medications (most notably the diuretics) must be avoided. Overproducers of uric acid (e.g., psoriasis, leukemia, certain anemias, certain solid tumors) should be treated with allopurinol. Underexcreters—the vast majority of cases—should respond to probenecid.

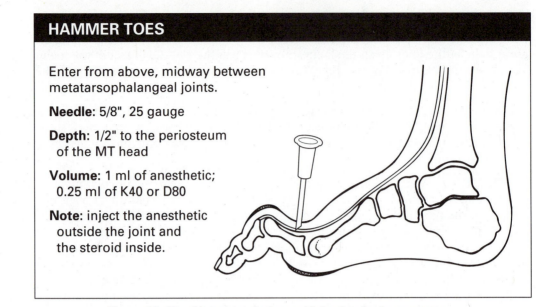

HAMMER TOES

Enter from above, midway between metatarsophalangeal joints.

Needle: 5/8", 25 gauge

Depth: 1/2" to the periosteum of the MT head

Volume: 1 ml of anesthetic; 0.25 ml of K40 or D80

Note: inject the anesthetic outside the joint and the steroid inside.

Figure 10–10.   Metatarsophalangeal injection for hammer toes.

Description   Hammer toes is the descriptive term used to describe the toe deformity caused by contracted extensor tendons in the foot. As the tendons slowly lose their flexibility, the MTP joints gradually extend and the proximophalangeal (PIP) joints gradually flex. The hammer-like deformity results. Pressure over these joints leads to plantar surface calluses and to dorsal surface corns (hypertrophic skin over the bony prominences).

Symptoms   The patient has pain over the toes, calluses, or abnormal-looking toes.

''My toes are crooked.''

''I can't bend my toes any more.''

''It's like walking on marbles. I have these thick calluses on the bottom of my feet.''

''The skin over the top of my toes is starting to thicken.''

''My toes are rubbing on my shoes.''

''It's hard to get shoes to fit.''

''At the end of the day my toes ache. The whole ball of my foot hurts.''

Exam   The extensor tendons are assessed for flexibility, the MTP joints are assessed for irritation and thickening, and the corns and calluses are documented.

EXAM SUMMARY

1. Tight extensor tendons
2. MTP joint tenderness
3. A positive MTP squeeze sign
4. Hammer toe deformity
5. Corns and calluses

(1) Regardless of the degree of hammer toe deformity, all patients have underlying tight or contracted extensor tendons of the foot. Forced plantarflexion of the MTP

joints and toes lead to tightness, pain, or both. This tightness may be experienced just over the dorsum of the foot or up the anterior surface of the leg. (2) Individual MTP joints may be tender. Tenderness is best elicited by compressing the joint from above and below and rolling the plantar MTP head between the fingers. (3) If the joints are particularly inflamed, the MTP squeeze sign will be painful. In this maneuver, all the joints are compressed simultaneously by side pressure (medial to lateral). (4) The typical hammer toe deformity is seen in well-established cases (p. 122). (5) Corns over the top of the PIP joints and calluses below the MTP joint are seen as the deformity progresses.

X-Rays   X-rays are not necessary for the diagnosis but are helpful in excluding other conditions. Patients with dramatic tenderness and swelling should have a radiograph to rule out rheumatoid arthritis. Patients with advanced cases may show degenerative changes at the MTP joints helpful in determining the prognosis. The typical hammer toe deformity is best seen on the lateral projection. Rheumatoid and degenerative arthritic changes are best seen on the anteroposterior view.

Diagnosis   The diagnosis is based on a history of pain over the balls of the feet and an exam showing localized metatarsal tenderness or the typical hammer toe deformity with normal radiographs. The diagnosis becomes confusing when the typical deformity is not present. These early cases are often labeled as metatarsalgia, a descriptive term used to describe any pain over the MTP joints. On close examination, the extensor tendons still show a loss of flexibility in flexion.

Treatment   The goal of treatment is to re-establish normal toe alignment by stretch exercises of the dorsal extensor tendons.

Step 1: Wide toe-box shoes are essential.
   Wear padded insoles to reduce the pressure over the metatarsal heads (p. 185).
   Use hammer toe crests (p. 187).
   Pare down the secondary corns and calluses.
   Use cotton or rubber spacers between the toes (p. 188).
   Do stretch exercises for the toes in plantarflexion.

Step 2 (4 to 6 weeks): Give a local injection of the MTP joints with D80.
   Re-emphasize the stretch exercises.

Step 3 (3 to 4 months): Consider surgical referral for flexor tenotomy or arthroplasty.

Physical Therapy   Physical therapy plays an important role in the active treatment and prevention of this problem. The focus of therapy is active stretching of the extensor tendons. After soaking the feet in warm to hot water for 15 minutes, the toes are held firmly at the MTP joints and the toes are passively flexed downward in the plantarflexion direction. Sets of 20 to 25 stretches are performed once a day. Initially, these sets are performed with the ankle and foot in the neutral position. As flexibility is restored, the ankle is plantarflexed more and more to accentuate the stretching. A pulling sensation should be felt in the anterior portion of the lower leg! Active stretching exercises are used to maintain flexibility. These exercises include curling the toes up and down, grasping the carpet, and picking up a small rolled towel.

Injection Technique   A local injection is used infrequently for this condition. Stretch exercises and padding are the principal treatments.

Position: The patient is placed in the supine position with the leg in extension and the foot plantarflexed.

Technique: The MTP joint is approached from the dorsal side. The MTP joint line is identified by gently subluxing the proximal phalangeal bone dorsally. This is 1 cm proximal to the web of the foot typically. A 25-gauge needle enters, is introduced midway between the MTP joints, and is advanced at a 45-degree angle down to the bone of the metatarsal head (typically ½" down). With the needle held flush against the bone, a small amount of anesthetic is injected followed by ¼ ml of K40 or D80.

Restrictions: Walking is limited for 3 days. Padding and use of wide toe-box shoes are continued for 30 days. Stretch exercises are resumed at 4 weeks.

Prognosis Early medical treatment for the "flexible hammer toe" is very successful. Stretch exercises performed regularly over a period of months will reduce the deformity. If the MTP and PIP joints are already rigid, surgery can be considered. The flexor tendons can be cut (flexor tenotomy) or combined with removal of the head of the proximal phalanx (arthroplasty).

MORTON NEUROMA

Enter from above, 1/4" distal to the metatarsophalangeal joint.

Needle: 5/8", 25 gauge

Depth: 1/2" to 5/8" (below the transverse metatarsal ligament)

Volume: 0.5 ml of K40

Note: this is identical to a digital block; the needle enters perpendicular to the skin

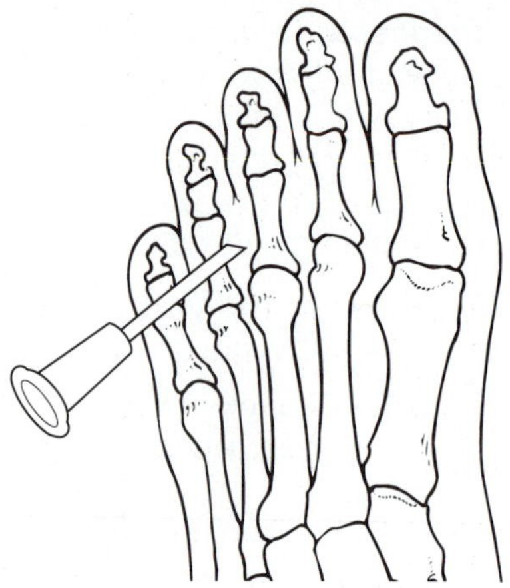

Figure 10–11.   Morton neuroma injection.

Description Morton neuroma is a chronic irritation/inflammation and enlargement of the digital nerve located in the web space between the metatarsal phalangeal heads. Pressure from below (walking or standing on hard surfaces with poorly padded shoes) and pressure from the sides (tight shoes) cause irritation and inflammation. Persistent pressure on the nerve for many months leads to enlargement characterized by perineural thickening and fibrosis.

Symptoms The patient has pain in between the toes or numbness of the sides of two adjacent toes.

"My two toes have gone numb."

"I have sharp pain between my toes."

"Certain tight shoes cause my toes to tingle."

"If I put all my weight on my right foot, I get a shooting pain through my toes."

"Sandals are the only shoes that feel comfortable."

"My third and fourth toes feel dead."

Exam Each patient should be examined for the degree of nerve irritation along with an assessment of neurologic function of the pair of digital nerves.

EXAM SUMMARY

---

1. Maximum tenderness is present in the web space
2. Loss of sensation along the inner aspects of the adjacent two toes (advanced case)
3. Pain aggravated by the MTP squeeze sign
4. Diagnostic nerve block

---

(1) Local tenderness is greatest in the web space between the MTP heads. This is in contrast to the tenderness at the MTP heads in metatarsalgia. Firm pressure is needed to elicit pain in the web space. (2) Pain can be reproduced by squeezing the MTP head from either side (medial to lateral). This compression may cause an electric-like pain to shoot to the ends of the adjacent two toes. (3) Advanced cases may show a loss of sensation along the inner aspects of the adjacent two toes. Light touch or pain sensation may be decreased.

X-Rays   X-rays are not necessary for the diagnosis. No characteristic changes are seen in the soft tissues. Calcification does not occur. The nerve enlargement is not great enough to cause erosion of bone.

Diagnosis   A presumptive diagnosis is based on the pain and local tenderness in the web space between two adjacent MTP joints. Confirmation of the diagnosis requires relief with local digital nerve block placed just below the transverse tarsal ligament. If the diagnosis is still in question and the patient's symptoms are unrelieved with conservative care, surgical exploration may be indicated for definitive diagnosis.

Treatment   The goals of treatment are to reduce the pressure over the nerve and to reduce the inflammation in the nerve.

Step 1: Wear wide toe-box shoes.
   Use padded insoles (p. 185).
   Use cotton or rubber spacer between the toes (p. 188).
   The NSAIDs are ineffective.

Step 2 (4 to 6 weeks): Give a local injection with K40.
   Re-emphasize the importance of proper shoes.
   Repeat the injection in 4 to 6 weeks if symptoms have not decreased by 50%.

Step 3 (3 months): Consider a referral to a podiatrist or orthopedist for a definitive neurectomy.
   Educate the patient, "Surgery will make the toes numb!"

Physical Therapy   Physical therapy does not play a significant role in the treatment of Morton neuroma.

Injection Technique   A local injection can be very effective when combined with treatment measures to reduce pressure.

Position: The patient is placed in the supine position with the leg held in extension and the foot slightly plantarflexed.

Technique: The nerve is approached from above. The proximal phalangeal heads are palpated. The 25-gauge needle is entered in the midline and advanced in a vertical position down through the transverse metatarsal ligament. A giving way can be felt when the needle passes through the ligament. One to 2 ml of anesthetic is injected, and the patient is re-examined. If the local tenderness between the phalangeal heads is relieved significantly, K40 is injected.

Restrictions: Walking and prolonged standing are restricted for 3 days. The recommendations for protection are continued for at least 2 months.

Prognosis Two consecutive injections with K40, 6 weeks apart, are effective in reducing the perineural inflammation around the digital nerve. The condition should be observed for at least 2 months prior to deciding on surgery. Nerve injuries take months to improve once the inflammation has been reduced and the offending irritation has been eliminated. A neurectomy can be considered for persistent symptoms. The patient should be informed that this leads to permanent numbness, because the entire nerve is removed.

SUMMARY

Local injection of corticosteroids is highly effective for both periarticular and articular conditions. Specifically, the *long-acting depot preparations* have been shown to be superior to the short-acting soluble preparations. Methylprednisolone acetate (Depo-Medrol) and either of the triamcinolone esters are the most concentrated, longest acting, and clinically most effective agents.

A variety of conditions have been shown to respond dramatically to local injection. It is the *treatment of choice* for trigger finger, de Quervain tenosynovitis, epicondylitis, and trochanteric bursitis. It may be superior to the nonsteroidal anti-inflammatory drugs (e.g., ibuprofen [Advil, Motrin]) for treating shoulder tendinitis, bursitis, and articular disorders involving the knee.

The overall response to injection is 80 to 90% and is greater in the upper extremity than in the lower weightbearing extremity. Five to 10% of disorders fail to respond to injection either because of tissue damage or disruption (mechanical dysfunction) or because of advanced disease (e.g., osteoarthritis). These cases often deserve surgical evaluation to exclude treatable mechanical problems or to set up for joint replacement.

Local injection is not without risk. The risk of *postinjection infection* is 1 to 6 per 10,000. *Atrophy* of the subcutaneous tissue or skin occurs in one third of cases but is limited to the soft tissues of the forearm and hand. *Postinjection inflammatory flare* also occurs in one third (especially with Depo-Medrol). This is self-limited and lasts for approximately 2 to 3 days. Ice will effectively control it. Lastly, the relationship of injection to *tendon rupture* remains controversial. Whether or not local injection causes tissue disruption, the four tendons that can rupture should be protected. Patients given injection for rotator cuff tendinitis or biceps tendinitis need to have a 30-day restriction of use. Patients given injection for Achilles tendinitis must wear a short-leg walking cast for 30 days. Patients given an injection for patellar tendinitis should wear a straight-leg brace for 3 to 4 weeks.

Ten Troublesome Fractures Commonly Encountered in Primary Care

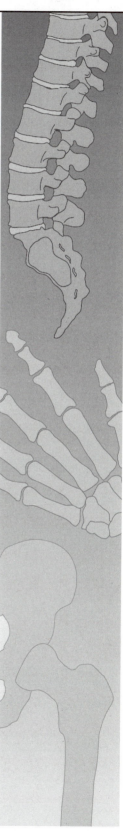

CHAPTER 11

Ten Troublesome Fractures Commonly Encountered in Primary Care

COMPRESSION FRACTURE OF THE SPINE

Evaluate for neurologic deficits and, in persistent cases, for posterior instability. Bedrest is suggested for 3 to 5 days. Narcotics are used liberally. Bowel care should be done. A complicating ileus should be kept in mind. Crutches are used after the acute pain has subsided. Hyperextension exercises and general lumbar spine stretches are begun as soon as pain lessens (p. 151). Surgery is indicated if angulation exceeds 35 degrees, if instability is present, or if the patient is neurologically compromised. A 3-point brace may be necessary to prevent flexion (>3 months). Healing takes 4 to 6 months.

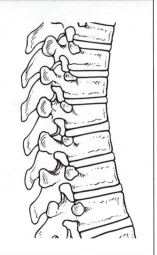

Figure 11–1. Vertebral compression fracture.

COLLES FRACTURE OF THE FOREARM

The entire forearm must be x-rayed to exclude elbow dislocation (Monteggia and Galeazzi lesions).
Anesthesia is used: hematoma, intravenous or regional arm block.
Reduction by traction and manipulation is performed to restore alignment and radiocarpal angulation.
A sugar-tong splint is applied (p. 174).
Arm elevation and ice are used for the first 24 to 48 hours. Active finger and shoulder exercises are begun in the first week.
Another x-ray is taken at 5 to 10 days and again in 4 to 6 weeks.

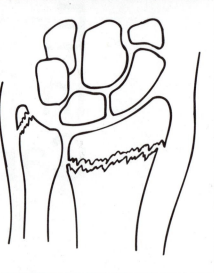

Figure 11–2. Colles fracture.

HUMERUS AND SURGICAL NECK FRACTURE

Immobilize with a shoulder immobilizer, a collar-and-cuff sling, or a sling-and-swathe bandage for 3 weeks (p. 169).
A hanging cast is rarely necessary (p. 170).
At 2 weeks, pendulum circumduction exercises are performed for 5 minutes, four times a day (p. 145).
Isometric toning exercises with a TheraBand should begin at 6 to 8 weeks (p. 146).
Total healing takes up to 12 weeks.
Surgical internal fixation is required when fragment displacement exceeds 1 cm or when angulation exceeds 45 degrees.

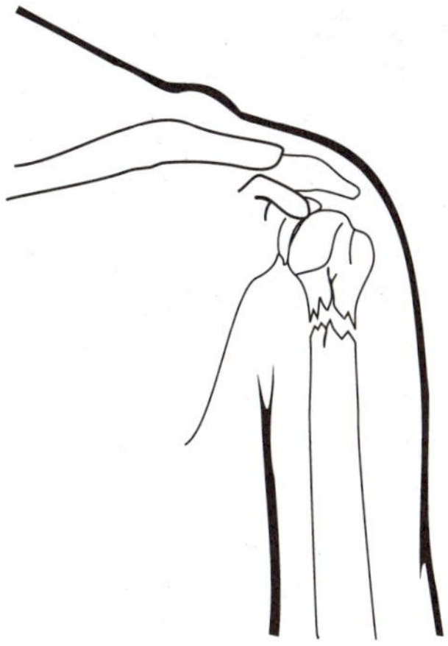

Figure 11–3.   Surgical neck fracture of the humerus.

FRACTURE OF THE CLAVICLE

Immobilization is the treatment of choice with a figure-of-eight (p. 170) splint, a shoulder immobilizer, or rarely a clavicular spica cast.
For a distal clavicular fracture, beyond the coracoclavicular ligament, a simple sling is sufficient (p. 169).
Surgery is rarely indicated, except for comminuted fractures; intramedullary pinning with a Knowles pin is the most common procedure.

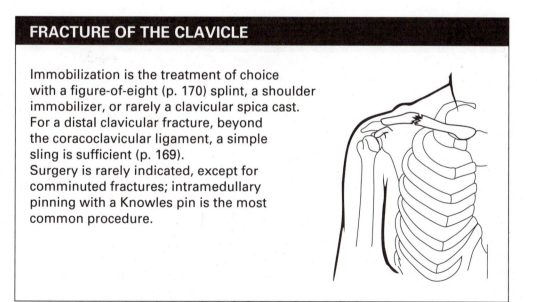

Figure 11–4.   Fracture of the middle third of the clavicle.

NAVICULAR FRACTURE

A high index of suspicion is necessary. Immobilization is mandatory when a sprained wrist is accompanied by local tenderness in the snuffbox or over the navicular, pain with grip is present, and motion of the wrist is decreased.
A thumb spica cast (p. 175) with 25 degrees of wrist extension and 20 degrees of radial deviation or an ant-post splint with an Ace wrap is used for 4 to 6 weeks. It may take 6 to 12 months for the fracture line to obliterate.
Surgery consists of bone grafting or Silastic arthroplasty.
The incidence of nonunion is 5 to 8%.

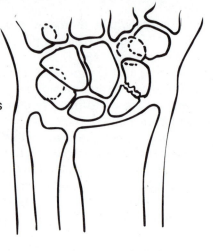

Figure 11–5.   Fracture of the navicular.

RIB FRACTURES

Uncomplicated rib fractures do not require special treatment. Hemothorax, pneumothorax, and flail chest must be watched for. Chest wall supports must be used cautiously: a large bra, a rib binder, or strapping with surgical tape can lead to pneumonia.
Pain medication and cough suppressants are useful but may lead to atelectasis or pneumonia. Healing takes 4 to 6 weeks. Surgery is reserved for complications only.

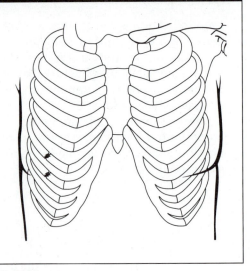

Figure 11–6.   Rib fractures.

HIP FRACTURE

The leg is shortened and rotated externally. Distinguish from a subcapital femoral neck fracture (more severe; requires surgical intervention!).
Bedrest with Buck traction 3 to 4 kg minimum, up to 6 kg plus medial and lateral straps.
Surgery for the osteoporotic elderly patient: compression screw fixation, Knowles pins, or Zickel nail fixation.
Medical follow-up for pneumonia, arrhythmia, subtle stroke, thromboembolism, coronary heart failure, etc.

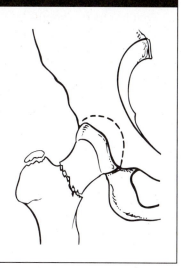

Figure 11–7. Intertrochanteric fracture of the hip.

TIBIAL STRESS FRACTURE

This fracture is seen almost exclusively in runners.
The results of plain x-rays can be normal in early cases.
Bone scans are much more sensitive, although a repeat x-ray in 2 to 3 weeks can be just as diagnostic.
Restrict running, jogging, and other impact exercises by at least 50% (DON'T try to convince a serious runner to stop running!).
Emphasize bicycling, swimming, and other non–weight-bearing sports.
An air cast is occasionally used (p. 183).
Medications have little effect.
Surgery is not indicated.

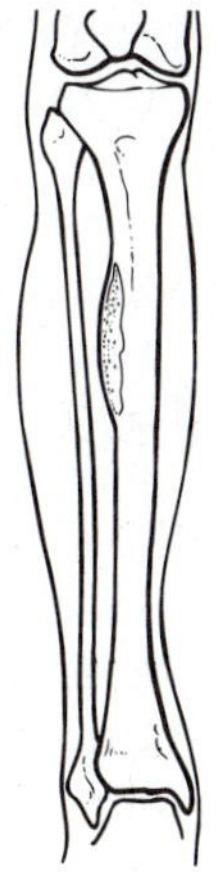

Figure 11–8. Midshaft tibial stress fracture.

CALCANEAL STRESS FRACTURE

This fracture is seen almost exclusively in runners.
The posterior third of the calcaneus is the site of
a bony fatigue fracture.
A repeat x-ray or bone scan is used to make
a diagnosis.
Padded insoles in well-fitting shoes are
suggested (p. 185).
A shortened stride may lessen some
of the heel strike pressure.
Running, jogging, and other high-
impact sports should be limited.
Emphasize non–weight–bearing
sports.

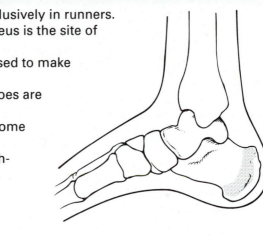

Figure 11–9.   Stress fracture at the heel.

MARCH FRACTURE

The metatarsals are tender, the dorsum of the
foot can be extremely edematous, and the
metatarsophalangeal or midfoot squeeze is
very painful.
The cortex of the metatarsal is thickened
on a plain x-ray.
Bone scanning can be used at presentation
to diagnose early cases.
Weightbearing must be reduced either by
reduced running, walking, or with crutches.
Wide toe box shoes are recommended.
Padded insoles will reduce some of the
discomfort (p. 185).
An air cast may be necessary for persistent
cases (p. 183).

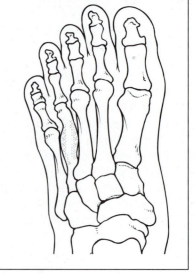

Figure 11–10.   Stress fracture of the metatarsal.

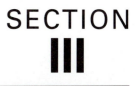

Exercise Instruction Sheets for Home Physical Therapy

Physical Therapy

Physical therapy is vitally important in the overall management of many of the local musculoskeletal conditions. Massage, stretching and toning exercises, ultrasound, phonophoresis, and thermal applications play a significant role in their recovery and rehabilitation. This is especially true for conditions that have a strong element of *mechanical dysfunction* when compared with the degree of inflammation. As examples, physical therapy treatments are very important in the treatment of subacromial impingement seen with rotator cuff tendinitis, in the treatment of the gait disturbance seen with trochanteric bursitis, and in the rehabilitation of the glenohumeral joint seen with frozen shoulder. All of these conditions have a unique mechanical component that requires specific physical therapy treatment for resolution.

In order to be effective without aggravating the underlying process, physical therapy treatments must be started at the appropriate *time* and at the appropriate *stage* of recovery. For example, stretch exercises to mobilize the ankle joint after a severe ankle sprain must be timed appropriately and performed in the proper sequence. Similarly, isometric toning of the rotator cuff tendons after rotator cuff tendinitis must be started at the appropriate time and begun at the suitable tension level. These recommendations cannot be predetermined with certainty. The decision to initiate any physical therapy treatment must be assessed by the primary care provider and should be based on (1) the phase of recovery, (2) the patient's ability and willingness to carry out a home exercise program, and most important, (3) the patient's tolerance of the specific exercise as determined by the health care provider in the office. Demonstration of the exercises in the office engenders greater confidence in the provider's treatment plan, provides hands-on explanation of the exercise, and allows the provider to assess the patient's understanding and tolerance of the exercise.

Nevertheless, guidelines for prescribing physical therapy do exist. General recommendations for treatment of joint conditions differ from those for the periarticular conditions. The following recommendations must be altered according to the criteria listed earlier. It cannot be overstated that the appropriateness of range of motion stretching, deep muscle massage, or isometric toning must be assessed individually on a case-by-case basis by physical exam and must be adjusted as the patient recovers.

Joint Conditions

1. Apply ice and elevate for acute pain and swelling.

2. Gentle range of motion stretching exercises can be performed during the acute phase of the condition, but only in the directions that are tolerated well or only to the point of mild discomfort.

3. Aggressive stretching exercises of the joint are appropriate 3 to 4 weeks after the acute injury, as long as this is tolerated clinically and the directions of motion will not incite further pain or inflammation.

Tendon and Ligament Conditions

1. Apply ice and elevate for acute pain and swelling.

2. Gentle range of motion stretching exercises of the affected joint should be started after the acute swelling and pain have resolved (after the estimated time it takes to heal microtearing, approximately 3 to 4 weeks). Initial stretching is performed in the directions that will not stretch the tendon or ligament directly.

3. If the affected joint has been immobilized for 2 to 3 weeks, range of motion stretching exercises are performed daily. A reasonable amount of joint mobility must be restored before resuming normal activities. The joint is preferentially stretched in directions that will not stretch the tendon or ligament directly.

4. After achieving reasonable flexibility (comparing side to side), isometric toning exercises of the supporting tendons are begun, followed by isometric toning of the affected tendon when stability has been significantly improved.

Bursal Conditions

1. Apply ice and elevate for acute swelling and inflammation.
2. Stretching exercises for tendons or ligaments that are responsible for the direct pressure over the bursa are begun as soon as the acute symptoms have resolved.
3. General stretching and toning of the adjacent joint is attempted.

GENERAL CARE OF THE NECK

Anatomy   The neck is made up of seven neck bones (vertebra) connected together by a network of ligaments and muscles, all of which serve to protect the spinal cord and the spinal nerves. Seven pairs of spinal nerves exit the spinal column and travel down the neck through the shoulder and into the lower arm. Each nerve must pass by one of the disks and through an opening (foramen) formed by two adjacent neck bones.

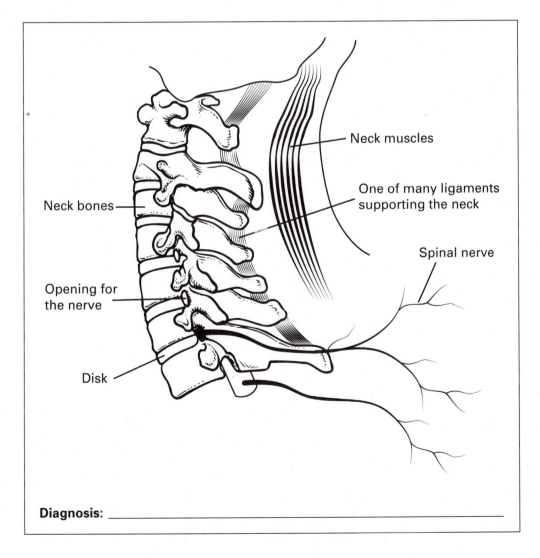

Neck muscles

One of many ligaments supporting the neck

Spinal nerve

Neck bones—

Opening for the nerve

Disk—

Diagnosis: _____

Conditions   Neck problems are exceedingly common. Everyone develops some degree of arthritis as they age, causing stiffness and lack of mobility (especially turning from side to side). Everyone at one time or another develops muscular irritation in the neck and upper back. Tension, emotional strain, and poor posture lead to cervical strain. Many patients suffer constant neck stiffness, headaches, and pain from whiplash injuries. Rapid deceleration injuries in a motor vehicle accident can cause permanent damage to the neck's supporting ligaments and muscles. Some patients develop symptoms down the arm from a pinched nerve. This can be caused by large bony spurs from arthritis (90%) or a herniated disk (10%), impairing spinal nerve function.

Physical Therapy   Physical therapy is fundamental to the treatment and prevention of conditions affecting the neck.

PHYSICAL THERAPY SUMMARY

1. Heat and massage
2. Neck muscle stretch exercises
3. Stress reduction
4. Ultrasound
5. Vertical cervical traction

Heat should be applied to the muscles of the neck prior to exercising. A shower, a hot bath, or a moist towel (warmed in a microwave) applied for 10 to 15 minutes is effective.

Massage is applied to either side of the neck and upper back muscles using hand pressure or an electric hand-held vibrator. The neck muscles should be relaxed during massage, either by supporting the head or by lying down.

Stretch exercises are used to increase flexibility and preserve motion (p. 142). Each exercise is performed in sets of 20, gradually increasing the stretch through the muscles. Mild discomfort is to be expected. Sharp pain or electric-like pain is a sign of excessive stretching or spinal nerve irritation.

Reduction in stress and improvement in *posture* help to reduce the tension and pressure in the neck. Upper back massage, gentle vibration with heat, relaxation techniques, or meditation may be very helpful in selected cases.

Ultrasound of the neck and upper back muscles can be combined with deep massage and stretch exercises. Neck strain and whiplash respond well to this combination.

Vertical cervical traction is reserved for chronic whiplash, chronic neck strain, and arthritis associated with a pinched nerve (see below). Vertical stretching of the neck muscles and ligaments must be started gradually and increased slowly.

Activity Limitations   These positions that emphasize a neutral neck position. The activities emphasize low levels of stress, protecting the muscles and ligaments and allowing gradual recovery.

Do not work overhead for long periods, especially looking up.
Do not sleep on the stomach with the neck turned or rotated.
Avoid stressful situations.
Do not go back-packing.
Avoid carrying heavy objects.
Avoid carrying a heavy purse over the shoulder.
Avoid continuous sitting.

Good Body Mechanics   These recommendations emphasize correct posture, neutral neck positions, and preventative measures.

Sit up with the shoulders back.
Sleep with the head aligned with the torso.
  On the back with a small pillow.
  On the side with enough pillows to keep the head straight.
Choose seat belts or an air bag.
Use the arm rests to keep the shoulders slightly shrugged.
Take periodic breaks from desk-top work.
Avoid continuous sitting or standing.
Choose a chair with good lumbar support.

Precautions   Stretch exercises are not always tolerated in patients with advanced arthritis with limited mobility or in patients with symptoms of a pinched nerve. Extremes of neck turning and neck extension can be painful and harmful, increasing the pressure over the nerve. Likewise, the deep heating and resultant swelling of ultrasound treatments may aggravate the symptoms associated with a pinched nerve. Vertical cervical traction must be used cautiously in patients with severe muscle irritation. Overly aggressive traction (too much weight or too long a period of traction) may aggravate the underlying muscular irritability.

STRETCH EXERCISES FOR THE NECK

Heat the neck and upper back in a bath tub, in a shower with a water massage, or with moist towels heated in a microwave. Gently stretch the muscles in sets of 10 to 15, with each held for 5 seconds. Expect mild, achy muscle pain but not sharp or electric pain. Relax the muscles in the neck during the exercises. Perform these exercises in the morning to relieve stiffness and just before sleeping.

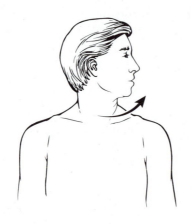

Neck Rotation
Slowly turn the head to the right. Place tension on the chin with the fingertips. Hold for a few seconds, and return to the center. Repeat to the left.

Neck Tilting
Tilt the head to the right, trying to touch the ear to the tip of the shoulder. Place tension on the temple with the fingertips. Hold for a few seconds, and return to the center. Repeat to the left.

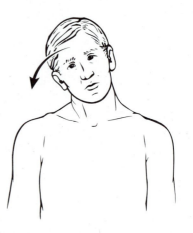

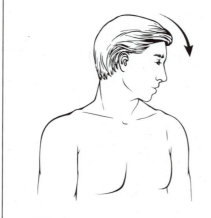

Neck Bending
Try to touch the chin to the chest. Hold for a few seconds, and return to the neutral position. Breathe in gradually, and exhale slowly with each exercise. Relax the neck and back muscles with each neck bend.

NECK MASSAGE

Heat the upper back and the neck for 15 minutes. Lie down on your stomach with your head aligned with your body. (Place a pillow under your chest and neck.) Ask your partner to press firmly with circular motions along the side of the neck and over the upper back muscles.

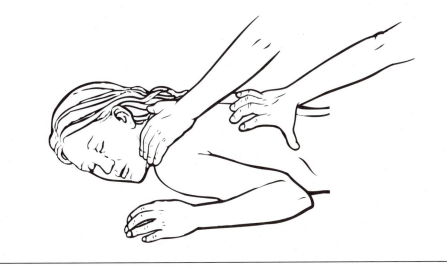

HOME CERVICAL TRACTION

Home traction using a cervical water bag traction unit can be started after an evaluation by a physical therapist. Traction is begun using 4 to 5 lb of water weight for 5 minutes and is slowly increased to 12 to 15 lb for 10 minutes. Each week, the weight and/or time is increased by 1 to 2 lb and/or 1 to 2 minutes. The neck muscles should be relaxed. Heat application prior to treatment is advised.
Note: Traction can aggravate some conditions, particularly some disk herniations. If symptoms worsen, stop the traction and re-evaluate. Arthritis of the neck may need to be treated three times a week for an indefinite period.

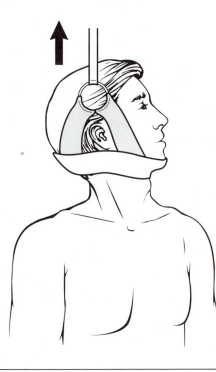

GENERAL CARE OF THE SHOULDER

Anatomy   The shoulder is a **ball-and-socket** joint formed by the upper arm bone (humerus), the cap of the shoulder (acromion process), and the bony socket (the glenoid of the scapula). It has many moving parts, including:

3 Separate joints	The ball and socket, the end of the collar bone (acromioclavicular joint), and the wing over the ribs (scapulothoracic)
7 Major tendons	4 rotator cuff tendons, biceps, triceps, and pectoralis
1 Major lubricating bursal sac	Subacromial
4 Major ligaments	3 over the end of the collar bone and 1 encircling the ball-and-socket joint

Conditions   There are many causes of shoulder pain, including pain from tense neck and upper back muscles, pain from a pinched nerve in the neck, shoulder strain or separation, tendinitis, bursitis, or arthritis. However, shoulder tendinitis of the rotator tendons and frozen shoulder from disuse account for two thirds of all problems.

Physical Therapy   Physical therapy plays a major role in the active treatment and rehabilitation of shoulder conditions.

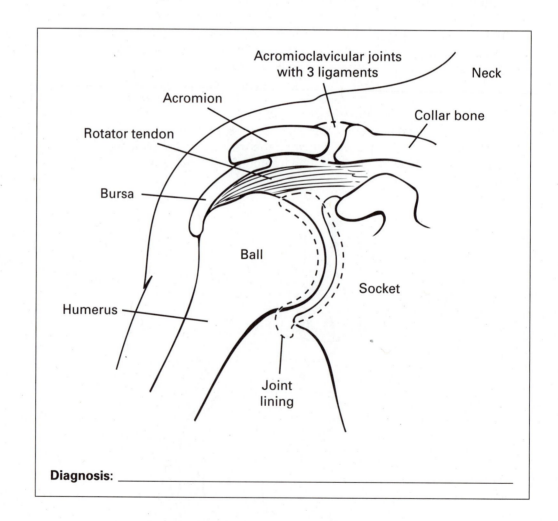

Diagnosis: _____

PHYSICAL THERAPY SUMMARY

1. Heat and massage
2. Weighted pendulum stretch exercises
3. Isometric toning exercises
4. Activity limitations
5. Stress reduction

FIRST FEW DAYS AND WEEKS   The shoulder is *heated* in a shower or warm bath for 10 to 15 minutes. Total body heating is preferred to local heat, using either a moist heating pad or a towel warmed in a microwave.

The *weighted pendulum exercise* is used to gently stretch the tendon space between the ball-and-socket joint and the cap (see below). A weight of 5 to 10 lb is held in the hand. A filled gallon milk jug weighs 8 lb, but any weight that can be easily hand-held will do. The arm is kept vertical and close to the body. The muscles of the shoulder are relaxed, allowing the weight to stretch out the tendon space. The exercise is performed after heating the shoulder for 5 minutes once or twice a day.

PENDULUM SWING EXERCISES FOR THE SHOULDER

Prior to exercise or heavy work, shoulders need to be stretched in a downward direction. This exercise provides greater space for the rotator cuff and the biceps tendons, allowing them to work more effectively and efficiently. Regular use of pendulum exercises can increase the space under the cap of the shoulder by 1/4".

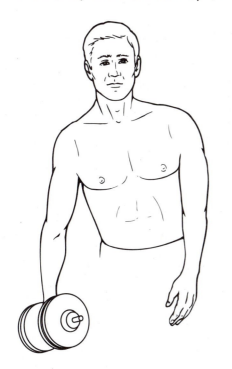

Weighted Pendulum Swings
Heat the shoulder with moist towels or in a hot bath or hot shower. A weight of 5 to 10 lb is held lightly in the hand (a filled gallon container weighs 8 lb). The muscles of the shoulder are relaxed! The arm is kept vertical and close to the body (bending over too far may cause pinching of the rotator cuff tendons). The arm is allowed to swing back and forth or in a small diameter circle (no greater than 1' in any direction).
A properly performed stretch exercise may cause a deep achy pain, either in the armpit or down the inner aspect of the arm. This exercise can be performed sitting just as effectively.

This exercise is very helpful for shoulder tendinitis (rotator cuff and biceps tendinitis), shoulder bursitis, frozen shoulder, and rotator cuff tendon tears. It is not appropriate for shoulder separation/strain or upper back/neck muscle strain.

RECOVERY/REHABILITATION *Isometric toning exercises* are used to strengthen the joint (see below). These should always follow the weighted pendulum stretch exercises. Rotation and lifting isometrics are performed in sets of 20, each held 5 seconds with moderate tension. Flexible rubber tubing, bungee cords, or large rubber bands provide the necessary resistance. These exercises are gradually increased to bring the weakened tendons and muscles into balance with the remaining tendons! Expect some mild soreness. Sharp or severe pain may indicate a flare of the underlying condition.

STRENGTHENING EXERCISES FOR THE ROTATOR CUFF TENDONS

The rotator cuff tendons are the weakest and most susceptible to injury of the seven major tendons at the shoulder. Isometric exercises are necessary to improve the strength of these tendons. These exercises will "balance" the strength of the shoulder muscles. Flexible rubber tubing, bungy cords, or large rubber bands are used to develop muscle tone and strength. First, the shoulder is heated and then prepared by stretching using the weighted pendulum swing exercise. Following a 2 to 3 minute rest, sets of 15 to 20 isometrics (each held 5 seconds) should be performed daily.

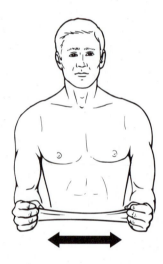

Rotation Isometric
The elbows are held at 90 degrees closely to the sides. The rubber bands are grasped with the hands. The forearms are rotated out 2 to 3" and held 5 seconds (forearms swing out like a door).

Lifting Isometric
The elbows are bent to 90 degrees. The rubber bands are placed near the elbows. The arms are lifted up 4 to 5" away from the body and held for 5 seconds.

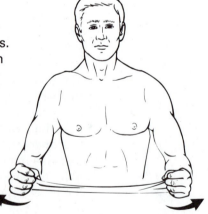

Note: These exercises are used for shoulder tendinitis, shoulder bursitis, and rotator cuff tendon tears and are begun 3 to 4 weeks after the acute inflammation has resolved. If begun too soon, these exercises may result in a flare up of the underlying condition! During the healing process, heavy work must be restricted!

146

Activity Limitations Activities and positions that require reaching out, up, or back are to be minimized:

Overhead reaching
Throwing
Sleeping with the arm overhead
Sleeping on the shoulder directly
Leaning on the elbows, jamming the shoulder
Lifting heavy objects with the arms extended
Heavy pushing and pulling
Serving and the overhead smash in tennis
Overhead military press
Incline bench press
Chin-ups and push-ups
Crawl and back strokes in swimming
Archery, pulling a 90-lb bow

Good Body Mechanics Safe activities and positions involve keeping the arm down, in front of, and close to the body.

Lifting objects close to the body
Weight training with light weights below the shoulder level
Side stroke or breast stroke
Side arm or underhand throwing
Volleying rather than serving
Desktop writing, assembly, and so forth, with good posture

Reductions in *stress* and improvements in posture help to reduce the pressure over the ball and socket and the shoulder tendons and bursa. Upper back and neck massage, gentle vibration with heat, relaxation techniques, or meditation may be very helpful in selected cases.

Precautions Weighted pendulum stretch exercises should be avoided if there is any history or suggestion of dislocation or partial dislocation of the ball-and-socket joint. Likewise, these exercises should be used with caution in patients with a history of shoulder separation at the acromioclavicular joint. Either condition can be aggravated by downward traction! Isometric toning exercises must be properly prescribed to be beneficial. Chronic shoulder tendinitis or shoulder tendinitis complicated by a torn tendon can be aggravated by overly aggressive toning. It is always safest to start out with low tension and to gradually increase the tension as tolerated!

STRETCH EXERCISES FOR A FROZEN SHOULDER

These exercises, performed once or twice a day for several months, should loosen the tightened shoulder lining and restore normal range of motion. First, heat the shoulder for 15 to 20 minutes and perform a 5 minute pendulum swing. Then, perform sets of 10 to 20 of the following three exercises. A mild muscle type pain along the front or side of the shoulder is expected. Severe discomfort is unusual and suggests overstretching.

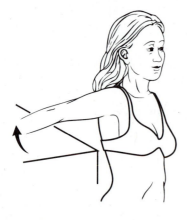

Armpit Stretch
Use your good arm to lift the arm onto a shelf, a dresser, or any object about breast high. Gently bend at the knees, opening up the arm pit. Try to push the arm up just a little bit further with each stretch.

Finger Walk Up The Wall
Face a wall at about three quarters of an arm's length. Using only your fingers (NOT your shoulder muscles) raise your arm up to shoulder level. Repeat this exercise.

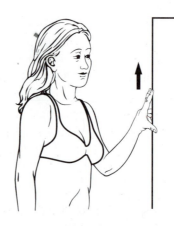

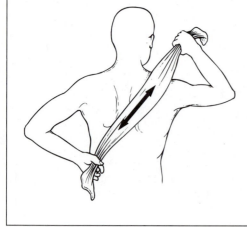

Towel Stretch Behind The Back
Take a 3' long towel, grasp it with both hands, and hold it at a 45 degree angle. Use the upper good arm to pull the arm toward the lower back. This can be repeated with the towel in the horizontal position.

TENNIS ELBOW STRENGTHENING EXERCISES

These exercises are begun 2 to 3 weeks after the acute pain and local tenderness have subsided. They strengthen the muscle and the tendon, reducing the risk of recurrent tendinitis. Muscle soreness in the forearm (2 to 3" down from the elbow) is common. If sharp or intense pain is felt in the outer elbow, the exercises should be discontinued (recurrence?).

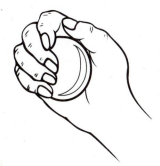

Grip Strengthening
Grip exercises should always precede wrist isometrics. Begin with a small compressible rubber ball (e.g., an old tennis ball, silicon ball). Grip firmly but not hard. Perform 20 to 25 mild squeezes, with each held for 5 seconds. With increasing strength, advance to a spring-loaded metal gripper.

Wrist Isometrics
After 2 to 3 weeks of grip exercises, isometric strengthening of wrist bending can be started. Perform 15 to 20 sets/day. Keep the wrist in a neutral position while pulling on a large rubber band, bungy cord, or flexible rubber tubing. Achy pain should be felt in the forearm, but sharp pain over the elbow may indicate recurrent tendinitis.

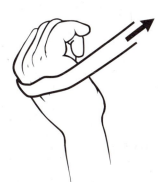

These exercises are preventive measures. In addition to these exercises, switch to a two-handed backhand, use power tools, wear a "tennis elbow band," try to lift objects with two hands, or emphasize lifting with the palms up.

STRETCHING OF THE WRIST AND HAND TENDONS

These stretch exercises help to rehabilitate and prevent trigger finger, thickened palms (Dupuytren), and carpal tunnel syndrome. They are begun 3 to 4 weeks after the acute pain and inflammation have resolved. The hand and wrist are heated for 15 to 20 minutes. The wrist and fingers are bent back using very light finger pressure.

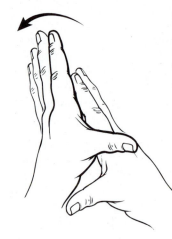

Wrist Stretching
Bend the wrist back as far as comfortable. Enhance the stretch with gentle constant tension against the fingers. A pulling sensation should be felt in the forearm. Perform sets of 15 to 20 per day.

Finger Stretching
Massage the palm and base of the fingers with Lanoline cream for 5 minutes. Stretch the affected fingers back with gentle finger pressure. Perform sets of 15 to 20 per day.

Gradual stretch exercises should be performed over several months to prevent a recurrence or to slow down the progression of the problem. In addition, avoid vibration tools, heavy gripping and grasping tools, and any tools that place pressure over the wrist or the palm tendons.

GENERAL CARE OF THE BACK

Anatomy   The lower back (lumbosacral spine) consists of **five back bones** (vertebra) connected together by a network of ligaments and muscles, all of which protect the spinal cord and spinal nerves. Five pairs of spinal nerves exit the spinal column and travel down the back through the pelvis and buttocks and into the lower leg. Each nerve passes by one of the spinal disks and through a bony passage formed by two adjacent back bones.

Conditions   Back problems are exceedingly common. Everyone will develop some degree of arthritis and at least one episode of low back strain. Poor posture, excessive weight, lack of exercise, and improper lifting all contribute to acute lumbar strain. Some patients develop symptoms down into the leg from a pinched nerve. The most common cause of a pinched nerve in the lower back is a herniated disk.

Physical Therapy   Physical therapy is essential to the treatment, rehabilitation, and prevention of low back conditions.

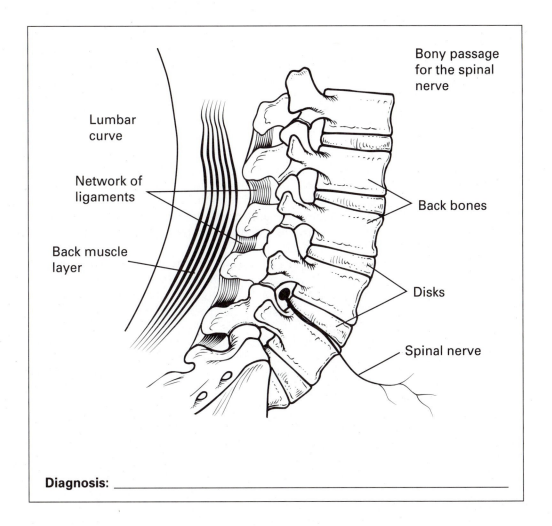

Diagnosis: _____

PHYSICAL THERAPY SUMMARY

1. Heat and massage
2. Cold for acute muscle spasm
3. Stretching exercises
4. Aerobic exercises (e.g., walking, swimming, cross-country ski machine)
5. Strengthening exercises
6. Vertical stretching
7. Ultrasound
8. Lumbar traction in bed
9. Chiropractic manipulation

FIRST FEW DAYS/WEEKS Cold, heat, massage, and gentle stretching exercises are used to treat the acute low back muscle irritation and spasm.

Cold, heat, or cold alternating with heat are effective in reducing pain and muscle spasm. Some patients respond to one better than another. A bag of frozen corn, an iced towel from the freezer, or an ice pack should be left in place for 15 to 20 minutes three to four times a day. Moist heat is preferred and is used similarly.

Massage of the lower back muscles is effective in reducing muscle spasm. This should always be performed on a comfortable surface while lying on the stomach. Hand pressure or pressure from an electric vibrator is applied from the lower rib cage to the top of the pelvis. Up-and-down and circular motions are performed on either side. This is especially effective just before going to bed.

Low back muscle *stretching exercises* are performed to restore lost flexibility. These exercises are especially important for patients suffering from scoliosis, compressed vertebra, or other structural back disorders. Side bends, knee-chest pulls, and pelvic rocks are designed to stretch the lower back muscles, the buttock muscles, and the sacroiliac joints (p. 153). These are begun after the most intense muscle spasms have resolved (usually days!). Initially, these should be performed in bed while lying down. As the pain and muscle spasm improves, stretching can be performed in the standing position. Sets of 20 of each exercise are performed to the point of mild muscular aching. Any sharp pain or any electric-like or shooting pain down the leg may be a sign of nerve irritation or overstretching!

Ultrasound treatments are used in selected cases. These require a physical therapist or chiropractor to administer. The device causes a vibration-like feeling but is actually heating the deep tissues. *Diathermy* is another special heat machine that provides deep heating. Both are used for difficult-to-treat muscle spasms. Patients with a herniated disk should avoid these treatments.

Chiropractic manipulation is an effective alternative to home physical therapy. Realignment by adjustment of the spinal elements has been shown to provide temporary benefit for acute lumbar strain. It is not appropriate to consider chiropractic treatments if there has been or there is serious consideration of a compression fracture, disk herniation, or disease of the bones of the back!

Patients failing to respond to the aforementioned acute treatments may require in-hospital *lumbar traction*. This type of treatment is rarely used today. Only the resistant cases of severe lower back muscle spasm would qualify. Several days of pelvic traction at 20 to 25 lb are combined with intense use of a strong muscle relaxant and narcotic medications.

RECOVERY/REHABILITATION Increasing degrees of stretching exercises are combined with toning exercises, aerobic exercises, and vertical traction to continue the recovery process and prevent a recurrence. These exercises are begun around 3 to 4 weeks after the acute symptoms have resolved.

Toning exercises of the abdominal and lower back muscles consist of modified sit-ups, weighted side bends, and gentle extension exercises (p. 156). These are always performed after heating and stretching (see later).

BACK STRETCHING EXERCISES

Back stretching exercises play a vital role in the treatment of lumbosacral muscle spasms. The lower back is heated for 15 to 20 minutes. Sets of 10 to 20 stretches, each held for 5 seconds, are performed on each side. The muscles are kept relaxed. Rest for 1 to 2 minutes between exercises. Mild muscle soreness is expected. Severe pain, electric-like sharp pain, or severe muscle spasms suggest overstretching.

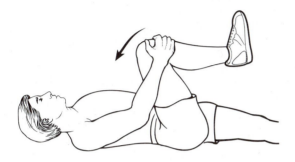

Knee-Chest Pulls
Bring the knee slowly up to the chest, holding it in place with the hands. Relax the buttock and back muscles. Do the left side, then the right side, and then both simultaneously (curling up in the fetal position).

Pelvic Rocks
With the knees bent, the pelvis is rotated forward and then backward. The abdominal muscles do the work as the back muscles are relaxed. CAUTION: do not overextend when arching the back!

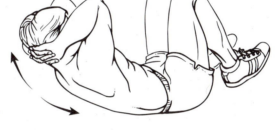

Side Bending
While lying down, crawl your fingers down the side of your thigh. Hold in this tilted position for 5 seconds. Return to a neutral position. Repeat on the other side.

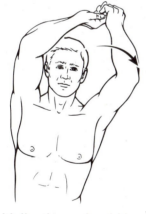

Initially, these should be performed while lying or while floating in the bath or hot tub. With improvement, these exercises can be performed standing or sitting. Follow these movements with exercises to strengthen the back (p.156).

Aerobic exercises are one of the best ways to prevent recurrent back strain. General toning of the body improves posture, muscular support, and flexibility. Swimming and cross-country ski machine work-outs are probably the best overall exercises that will not aggravate the back. Swimming, in particular, is an excellent way to recover lost muscular tone and function after a herniated disk, compression fracture, or spinal surgery. Fast walking and light jogging are acceptable forms of exercises also. Exercise apparatus that places excessive bend or torque in the back should be avoided.

Vertical traction can be used at home as a part of a comprehensive back treatment program (see below). The weight of the lower body and legs is used to pull the lumbar segments apart. Leaning against a countertop, suspending the body between two bar stools, or using inversion equipment for 1 to 3 minutes at a time will allow the back bones, ligaments, and muscles to gradually stretch out. Several vertical stretches are performed each day. It is extremely important to relax the whole lower body when performing this exercise and to slowly return to full weightbearing by lowering down to the legs very gradually.

ADVANCED BACK STRETCHING EXERCISES

This exercise is not appropriate for everyone. A strong upper body is a prerequisite as well as a 2 to 4 week period of basic back exercises (see pp. 153–156). The vertical stretch elongates the support ligaments, lengthens the back muscles, and allows the back bones to pull apart and realign. (I refer to this exercise as "the poor man's chiropractic adjustment.") Suspension between parallel bars is ideal, but any method to allow the weight of the legs to pull down on the back will work (e.g.,leaning on a countertop, crutches, supporting your weight between two bar stools).

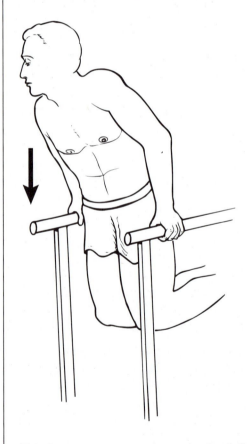

Vertical Stretch Exercise
Starting in a standing position, the weight of the body is gradually shifted to the outstretched arms. The toes are kept on the ground for balance. The back muscles should be relaxed. Allow the weight of the legs to draw-pull out the lower back bones. Popping sensations or a gentle sensation of stretch should be felt in the lower back. Additional pull occurs if you lean forward slowly. Hold this position for 30 to 60 seconds. Gradually shift the weight back to the legs and then stand up straight. Repeat once or twice. This exercise is especially helpful before going to bed.

This is a great way to keep the back limber and the back muscles supple. This exercise can be performed daily to prevent recurrent back strain.

For chronic cases that do not respond to traditional physical therapy, a transcutaneous electric nerve stimulator (TENS) unit can be tried along with a thorough evaluation by a pain clinic.

Activity Limitations   These positions and activities place excessive load or torque on the muscles, ligaments, and bones of the back:

Lifting heavy objects

Lifting objects away from the body (the arms held out)

Lifting in a twisted position

Working in a stooped position

Bending excessively at the waist

No full sit-ups

No bending over to touch the toes (at least in the recovery period)

Avoid the rowing machine, heavy weightlifting, or any apparatus that either puts too much bend, torque, or pressure into the lower back

Good Body Mechanics   These positions and activities are safest and reduce the possibility of reinjuring the muscles and ligaments:

Sitting and standing up straight

Lifting with the legs and knees

Lifting and carrying weight close to the body

Lifting using a external lumbar support

Sleeping on a firm mattress with a pillow under the knees

Keep the weight down

Wear seat belts and purchase a car with an air bag

Low weight, high repetition weightlifting

Swimming, cross-country ski machine (with low tension arm setting to avoid back twisting or torque), a soft platform treadmill, or fast walking

Precautions   Stretching and toning exercises should always be started gradually. If any sharp pain or electric-like pain or shooting pains down the leg occur, the exercises will have to be stopped. These symptoms suggest nerve irritation!

Ultrasound treatments should be avoided in patients with herniated disks. Deep heating may cause the disk to swell further!

Chiropractic manipulation must be avoided with bony compression fractures, disk herniations, and disease of the back bones!

Vertical traction must be used with caution. You must possess strong upper body strength and be free of cardiovascular disease (blood can pool in the legs and lead to fainting). Your health care provider should be contacted before starting this type of aggressive stretching.

BACK STRENGTHENING EXERCISES

Before starting a strengthening program for the back, flexibility must be restored with 3 to 6 weeks of daily back stretching. Strengthening exercises should be performed when the body is well rested. First, the back muscles are stretched out for 5 to 10 minutes (see p. 153). Then, sets of 15 to 20 of the following are performed daily for 6 weeks. As the strength of the back increases, the frequency can be reduced to three times a week.

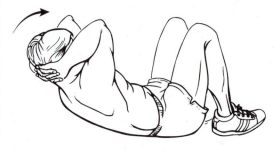

Modified Sit-ups
The knees are kept bent. The lower back is kept flush with the ground. The hands can be kept either behind the neck or held over the chest. The head and neck are raised 3 to 4" and held for 5 seconds. The abdominal muscles will gradually strengthen.

Weighted Side-bends
In a standing position, a 5 to 15 lb weight is held in the hand. The back is tilted to the weighted side and is immediately brought back to center. The back needs to be tilted only a few inches! The farther away from the body the weight is held, the greater is the amount of muscle work! After a set of 15 to 20, the weight is switched to the opposite side.

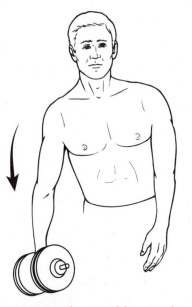

These specific exercises are complementary to a regular aerobic exercise program. No single exercise is better than another. If you are having problems doing any specific exercise, discuss it with your health care provider.

STRETCH EXERCISES FOR ARTHRITIS

Home physical therapy for hip arthritis consists of stretching and strengthening exercises. First, the hip is heated in a hot tub bath or with moist heat for 20 minutes. Then 15 to 20 knee chest, figure-of-four, and Indian-style exercises are performed to stretch the muscles and ligaments around the hip. After relaxing for 5 minutes, weighted straight leg raises and leg extensions are performed to strengthen the hip (see knee exercises, p. 161).

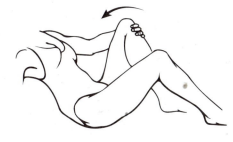

Knee-Chest Pulls
Bend the hip and knee to 90 degrees. Grasp the upper shin, and pull the knee onto the chest. Hold this position for 5 seconds, and then relax back to 90 degrees. These exercises should be performed lying down.

Figure-of-Four Stretch
The foot is placed over the knee. The leg is gently rocked outward. The higher the foot is raised on the leg, the greater is the stretch. Perform this exercise while lying down.

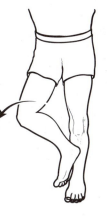

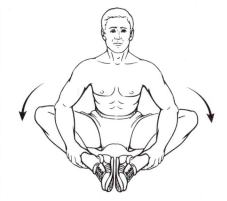

Indian Sitting Stretch
In a seated position, pull the feet up toward the buttocks. Lean forward gradually to increase the stretch.

STRETCH EXERCISES FOR HIP BURSITIS

The large buttock tendon over the outer hip needs to be stretched to reduce the pressure over the bursal sac. First, the area is heated either in a bathtub or with moist heat. Sets of 15 to 20 stretches are performed daily. Begin these 2 to 4 weeks after the outer hip pressure pain has resolved.

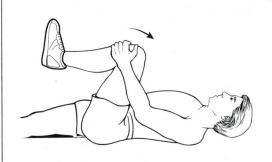

Knee-Chest Pulls

Bend the hip and knee to 90 degrees. Grasp the upper shin, and pull the knee onto the chest. Hold this position for 5 seconds, and then relax back to 90 degrees. A gentle pulling sensation should be felt in the buttock and low back area. These exercises are best performed while lying down but can be performed in a partially reclining position.

Cross-Leg Pulls

In a sitting position, either in chair or sitting on the floor, cross the affected leg over the other leg. Grasp the knee, and pull the leg to the opposite side. Keep the buttocks flat, and avoid twisting the back. A gentle pulling sensation should be felt in the outer buttocks or hip areas. Sharp pain suggests irritation of the bursa.

GENERAL CARE OF THE KNEE

Anatomy.   The knee is a **hinge joint** joining the thigh bone (femur), the lower leg bone (tibia), and the knee cap (patella). It has many moving parts including:

3 Joint compartments	Inner (medial), outer (lateral), knee cap (patellar)
2 Major muscle groups	Thigh muscle (quadriceps), back of the leg (hamstrings)
2 Hinge ligaments	Inner (medial collateral) Outer (lateral collateral)
5 Lubricating bursal sacs	Prepatellar, infrapatellar, suprapatellar, anserine, and Baker cyst
2 Shock-absorber cartilages	Inner (medial) and outer (lateral) meniscus

Conditions   Any of the parts of the knee can wear out, suffer injury, or become inflamed by overuse. However, irritation of the undersurface of the knee cap and wear-and-tear arthritis are the most common (nearly two thirds of all).

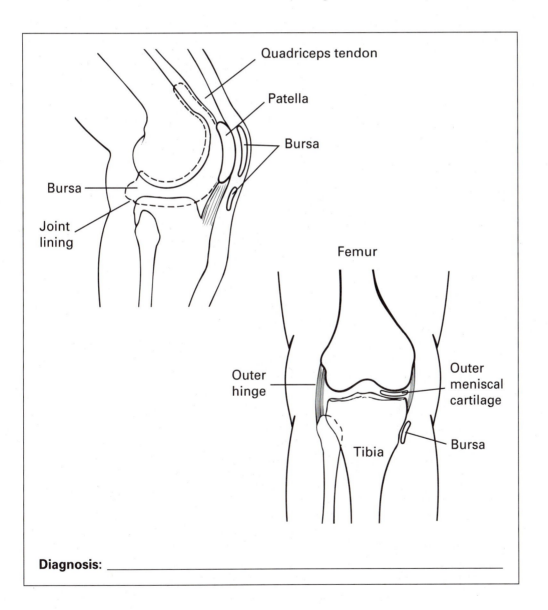

Diagnosis: _____

Physical Therapy   Physical therapy plays a very important role in the treatment of the variety of conditions that affect support structures of the knee and in the rehabilitation of the injured joint. Specific exercises are fundamental in improving knee support and stability.

PHYSICAL THERAPY SUMMARY

> 1. Ice
> 2. Ice + elevation
> 3. Straight leg raise and leg extension exercises
> 4. Activity limitations
> 5. Proper exercises and equipment

Ice is useful for the control of pain and swelling. Ice is applied for 15 to 20 minutes as often as every 2 to 4 hours. A bag of ice, a bag of frozen corn, or an iced towel cooled in the freezer work well.

Ice and elevation are indicated for the acutely swollen knee. The knee should be kept above the level of the heart.

Rehabilitation of the knee begins with gentle toning exercises. *Straight leg raise* and *leg extension* exercises are used to strengthen the quadriceps and hamstring muscles, to provide support to the joint, and to counteract the "giving-out" sensation caused by disuse (p. 161). Begin with sets of 10 leg lifts and gradually work up to 20 to 25 lifts, with each held 5 seconds. At first these are performed without weight, but with improvement weight is added to the ankle. Start with a 2-lb weight (e.g., a heavy shoe, fishing weights in a sock, a purse with a large book) and with improvement increase to a weight of 5 to 10 lb. Twisting and rotating the leg must be avoided. To secure the leg in the straight position, cock the ankle up!

Activity Limitation   These positions and activities place excessive pressure on the knee joint and must be limited until the pain and swelling resolves:

Squatting
Kneeling
Twisting and pivoting
Repetitive bending (e.g., stairs, getting out of a seated position, clutch and pedal
    pushing)
Jogging
Jazzercize
Stop-and-go sports (rackets and basketball)
Swimming with the frog or whip kick
Bicycling

Equipment Limitations   These types of exercise equipment place excessive pressure on the knee joint and must be limited until the pain and swelling resolves:

Stairstepper
Stationary bicycle
Rowing machine
Universal gym utilizing leg extensions

Acceptable Activities and Limitations   These activities place much less tension on the knee by limiting impact and repetitive bending:

Fast walking
Water aerobics
Swimming using the crawl stroke
Cross-country ski-glide machines
A soft platform treadmill
Trampoline

Weight loss is an issue in the long term!

KNEE STRENGTHENING EXERCISES

Nearly all conditions that affect the knee cause loss of tone in the thigh muscles (quadriceps and hamstrings). The strength of these muscles must be restored to restore knee stability.

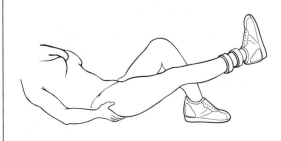

Straight Leg Raises

While sitting on the edge of a chair or while lying down with the opposite leg bent, the leg is raised 3 to 4" off the ground. Sets of 15 to 20 leg raises (each held for 5 seconds) are performed daily. Bending the knee should be avoided. After 2 to 4 weeks, the exercises are performed with a 5 to 10 lb weight placed at the ankle (e.g., a sock with fishing weights, an old purse with a large book, Velcro ankle weights).

Leg Extensions

While lying on the stomach or while up on all fours, the leg is raised perfectly straight 3 to 4" off the ground. Sets of 15 to 20 extensions (each held 5 seconds) are performed daily. After 2 to 4 weeks, the exercise is performed with a 5 to 10 lb weight added to the ankle. **Note:** This exercise must be performed while lying flat if the knee cap is the source of knee irritation!

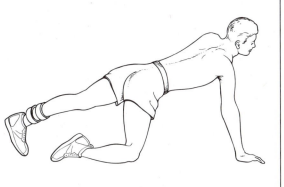

GENERAL CARE OF THE ANKLE

Anatomy   The ankle is a hinge joint that allows up and down bending and in and out turning of the foot. It is held together by a network of ligaments and supported by five major tendons. To function normally, the ankle must be properly aligned with the lower leg, must have intact and strong ligaments, and must have flexible and well-toned tendons.

Conditions   The most common condition affecting the ankle is the common ankle sprain. Injuries onto a turned-in ankle cause a separation or a tear of the supporting ligaments. Turned-in ankles associated with flat feet is a common problem that lead to an inflammation of the arch ligament (plantar fasciitis). Tendinitis at the ankle most commonly affects the Achilles tendon, which is located behind the ankle. Arthritis and bursitis at the ankle are not common.

Physical Therapy   Physical therapy plays an important role in the active treatment and rehabilitation of ankle conditions.

PHYSICAL THERAPY SUMMARY

1. Ice and elevation for acute swelling and pain
2. Heating before stretching
3. Stretching exercises especially for the Achilles tendon
4. Isometric toning exercises of inner and outer tendons

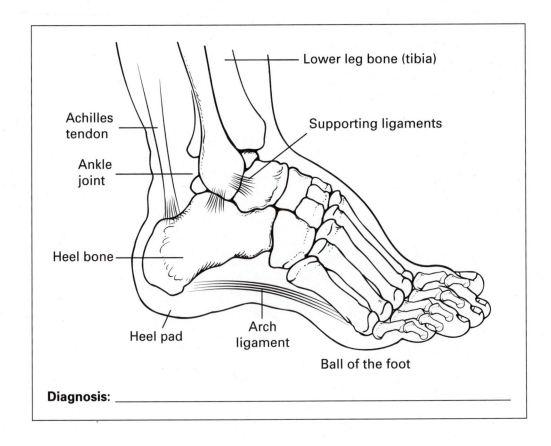

Diagnosis: _____

Ice and elevation of acute sprains, tendinitis, and joint swelling are always recommended for temporary relief of pain and swelling.

Heat is commonly recommended for recurrent or chronic ankle conditions requiring stretching and toning exercises. Heating provides additional blood flow and facilitates stretching.

Stretch exercises are commonly used to treat and rehabilitate Achilles tendinitis and the inflammation of the arch ligament (see below). These should always be preceded by heating for 10 to 15 minutes. Stretching exercises should be carried out over many weeks to avoid aggravating the underlying condition. Successful stretching should gradually improve over weeks.

ACHILLES TENDON STRETCH EXERCISES

Rehabilitation for Achilles tendinitis involves a long period of protection and gradual stretch exercises. Four weeks after the swelling and inflammation have resolved, the tendon is gradually stretched. The ankles are heated in water for 15 to 20 minutes. For the first 5 to 7 days, the ankle is pulled up by hand in sets of 20. With progress, the following two active exercises are performed.

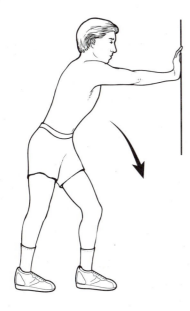

Wall Stretch
Face the wall and place your outstretched arms on the surface. Keep the affected leg behind. Partially flex the unaffected leg. While keeping the affected foot flat on the ground, gently lean forward. A pulling sensation should be felt in the calf, below the knee. Keep all of your body weight on the front leg!

Toe-Ups
The balls of the feet are placed on a 3" block or on the edge of the stairs. The muscle is tightened by tiptoeing. Then the muscle is relaxed and allowed to stretch when the heel drops below the level of the block. Do sets of 20 exercises.

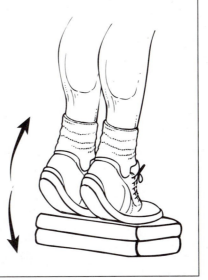

Isometric toning exercises are the most important means of improving ankle stability, weakened by disuse or injury (per below). Large rubber tubing, a TheraBand, or large rubber bands are used to gradually build up the tone and tension in the lower leg muscles. Each direction of ankle motion (bending up and down and turning in and out) are individually toned. As the stability of the ankle improves, the ankle braces can be gradually withdrawn.

Activity Limitations   These activities place too much tension across the supporting ligaments and tendons of the ankle:

> Running and jogging
> The stop-and-go sports (e.g., racketball, tennis, basketball)
> Jazzercize
> Trampoline
> Stairstepper
> Stair climbing with the ball of the foot
> Repetitive pedal use (e.g., clutch, heavy equipment)

ANKLE ISOMETRIC TONING EXERCISES

Isometric toning exercises of the ankle tendons are indicated for strengthening and stabilizing the ankle after disuse, injury, or immobilization. Large rubber tubing, a bungy cord, or large rubber bands are used to tone the lower leg muscles. Heating and stretching are performed prior to toning.

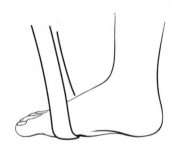

Achilles Tendon Toning
The rubber tubing is placed under the ball of the foot. The ankle is held steady at 90 degrees (a right angle!). The rubber tubing is pulled up by hand pressure and held for 5 seconds. Sets of 20 are performed daily.

Peroneus Tendon Toning
The rubber tubing is placed around the outside of each foot, next to the little toes. The ankle is held steady at 90 degrees (a right angle!). The legs are pulled apart 2 to 3" while holding the ankle firm for 5 seconds. Sets of 20 are performed daily.

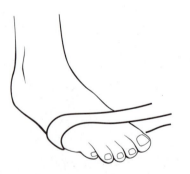

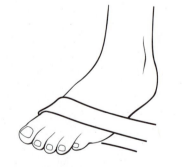

Posterior Tibialis Toning
The rubber tubing is placed around the inside of the foot next to the great toe and secured to a fixed object. The ankle is held steady at a 90-degree angle as the leg is pulled in toward the other. Sets of 20 (each held for 5 seconds) are performed daily.

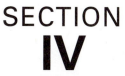

The Most Commonly Used Supports, Braces, and Casts

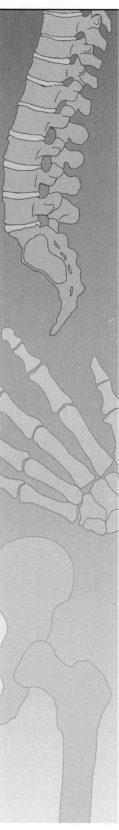

CHAPTER 13

Supports, Braces, and Casts

NECK

Soft Cervical Collar
Use: Cervical strain, whiplash, fibromyalgia,
  tension headaches
Advantage: Inexpensive, easy to put on,
  reasonably comfortable
Disadvantage: Doesn't restrict neck
  motion sufficiently
Cost: $4–5

Philadelphia Collar
Use: Neck trauma transport, herniated disk,
  postoperative recovery
Advantage: Much improved restriction of
  neck motion, some vertical stretch
Disadvantage: Cost; uncomfortable;
  slightly more difficult to put on
Cost: Soft—$35–40
  Hard—$60–65

Water Bag Cervical Traction
Use: Cervical radiculopathy, cervical strain, whiplash, fibromyalgia
Cost: $40–45

Pulsating Water Massager/Electric Hand Massager
Use: Cervical strain, tension headaches
Cost: $35–45

SHOULDER

Simple Shoulder Sling
Use: Acute bursitis, acute tendinitis, glenohumeral dislocation, acromioclavicular separation
Fractures: Postoperative recovery, surgical neck fracture
Advantage: Inexpensive; easy to put on; can be made at home
Disadvantage: Insufficient immobilization; can lead to frozen shoulder
Cost: $4–7

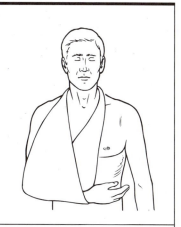

Abduction Pillow Shoulder Immobilizer
Use: Rotator cuff tendon tear, recovery from a rotator cuff surgery
Advantage: Excellent immobilization in a position of abduction
Disadvantage: Hard to put on; can lead to frozen shoulder; expensive
Cost: $40–42

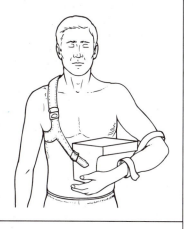

Sling and Swathe Bandage
Use: Glenohumeral dislocation, severe acromioclavicular separation
Fractures: upper humerus
Advantage: Better control of motion and pain; inexpensive
Disadvantage: Requires a technician; can't be removed easily by the patient
Cost: $4–5

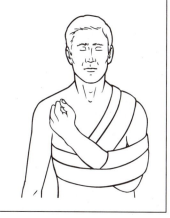

SHOULDER (cont.)

Shoulder Immobilizer
Use: Acromioclavicular separation, glenohumeral
  dislocation
  Fractures: humeral neck
Advantage: Easy to put on; relatively
  inexpensive; much less bulky; can be
  worn under clothing
Disadvantage: None
Cost: Universal—$19–22
  Velcro—$31–33

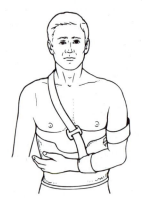

Figure-of-Eight Strap
Use: Acromioclavicular separation,
  glenohumeral dislocation
  Fractures: clavicle
Advantage: Inexpensive; easy to apply;
  can be worn under clothing
Disadvantage: Axillary irritation
Cost: $11–12

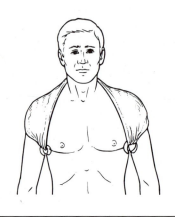

Hanging Cast
Use: No medical orthopedic indications
  Fractures: humeral surgical neck, humeral
  shaft fracture
Advantage: Provides downward traction on
  the fractured elements
Disadvantage: Heavy and bulky compared
  with a simple sling; more expensive;
  uncomfortable; requires a technician
Cost: $40–50

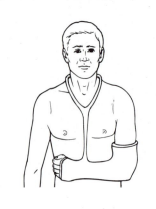

ELBOW

Tennis Elbow Band
Use: Lateral epicondylitis, extensor carpi radialis strain,
 brachioradialis strain
Advantage: Decreases the tension coming back
 to the tendon; inexpensive; easy to put on;
 not very restrictive
Disadvantage: Does not decrease
 the aggravation resulting
 from wrist use; probably only
 works for mild cases
Cost: $8–12

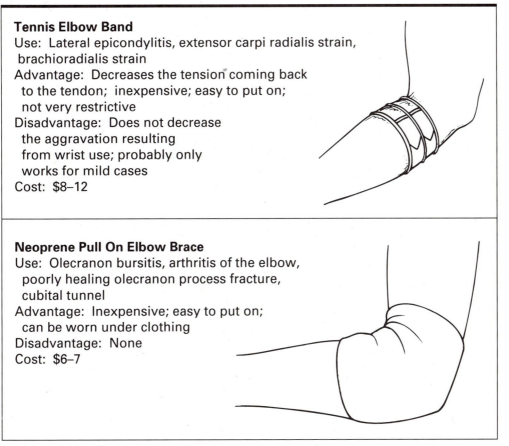

Neoprene Pull On Elbow Brace
Use: Olecranon bursitis, arthritis of the elbow,
 poorly healing olecranon process fracture,
 cubital tunnel
Advantage: Inexpensive; easy to put on;
 can be worn under clothing
Disadvantage: None
Cost: $6–7

WRIST

Simple Velcro Wrist Support
Use: Sprained wrist, weightlifting support
  Fractures: carpal bones, healing phase
Advantage: Inexpensive; lightweight;
  easy to put on
Disadvantage: Very little wrist
  support or restriction in wrist
  motion
Cost: $6–7

Velcro Wrist Immobilizer With Metal Stays
Use: Lateral and medial epicondylitis, carpal tunnel syndrome,
  severe wrist sprains, radiocarpal arthritis, dorsal ganglion
Advantage: Good restriction of wrist motion;
  relatively inexpensive; light
  weight, easy to put on
Disadvantage: Can cause
  pressure over the thumb
  and a temporary numbness
  of the local cutaneous nerve;
  may not restrict wrist motion sufficiently for specific condition
Cost: $17–18

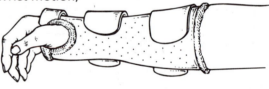

Short Arm Cast
Use: Lateral and medial
  epicondylitis, metacarpal
  subluxation
  Fractures: Colles, navicular,
  miscellaneous forearm fractures
Advantage: Best support and
  restriction of the wrist; cannot be
  removed
Disadvantage: Bulky; heavy; susceptible to
  water damage; more expensive; not universally
  available; requires a technician
Cost: Plaster— $25–27; fiberglass— $45–47

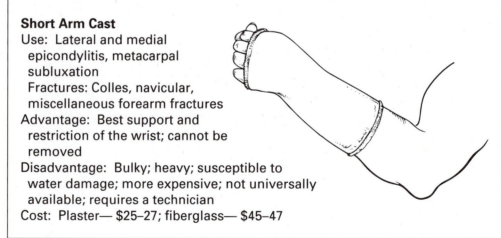

WRIST (cont.)

Radial Gutter Splint
Use: Fractures: nondisplaced metacarpals
   No. 2 and 3 and nondisplaced
   No. 1 and 2 phalanges
Advantage: Lighter weight than
   a short arm cast; can be removed,
   more convenient
Disadvantage: Can be removed,
   interfering with healing;
   insufficient immobilization
Cost: Plaster—$21–23; fiberglass—$39–40

Dorsal Hood Splint
Use: de Quervain tenosynovitis
   carpometacarpal arthritis
Advantage: Removable;
   lightweight
Disadvantage: Requires a
   technician; not as durable
   as the Velcro splints
Cost: Plaster—$15–16;
   fiberglass—$28–30

Ulnar Gutter Splint
Use: Ulnar collateral ligament strain, triangular cartilage injuries
   Fractures: Boxer's, nondisplaced No. 4 and 5 phalanges
Advantage: Removable; lightweight
Disadvantage: Requires a technician;
   not as durable as the Velcro splints
Cost: Plaster—$21–23;
   fiberglass—$39–40

WRIST (cont.)

Sugar-tong Splint
Use: Fractures: Colles, distal radius
  (Note: temporary splints only!)
Advantage: Allows swelling in first few days;
  easy to recheck the fracture
Disadvantage: Insufficient
  immobilization compared
  with a short arm cast;
  expensive to put two casts on
Cost: Plaster—$35–37;
  fiberglass—$65–67

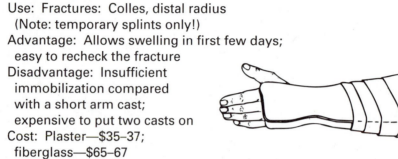

Padded Shell Velcro Thumb Splint or Velcro Thumb Spica Splint
Use: Carpometacarpal arthritis, de Quervain tenosynovitis,
  gamekeeper's thumb
Advantage: Lightweight;
  comfortable; relatively
  inexpensive
Disadvantage: May not
  sufficiently restrict motion
Cost: $25–28

Thermoplastic Molded Thumb Splint
Use: Carpometacarpal arthritis, gamekeeper's thumb
Advantage: Custom fitted; excellent support
  and immobilization
Disadvantage: Requires a technician;
  may be overly limiting to the
  patient
Cost: $25–26

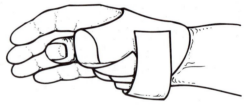

WRIST (cont.)

Taping for Osteoarthritis of the Thumb
Use: Carpometacarpal arthritis, gamekeeper's thumb
Advantage: Very inexpensive; permits
  some use without much aggravation;
  can be applied by the patient
  whenever needed
Disadvantage: Doesn't last; must be
  reapplied; easily soiled
Cost: $1–2

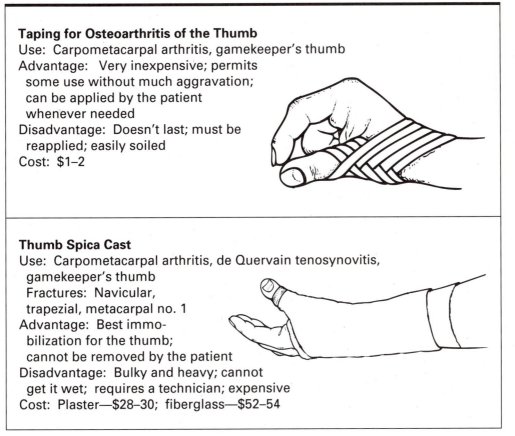

Thumb Spica Cast
Use: Carpometacarpal arthritis, de Quervain tenosynovitis,
  gamekeeper's thumb
  Fractures: Navicular,
  trapezial, metacarpal no. 1
Advantage: Best immo-
  bilization for the thumb;
  cannot be removed by the patient
Disadvantage: Bulky and heavy; cannot
  get it wet; requires a technician; expensive
Cost: Plaster—$28–30; fiberglass—$52–54

HAND

Buddy Taping

Use: Simple finger sprains,
  trigger finger, osteoarthritis of
  the finger joints, de Quervain
  tenosynovitis
  Fractures: nondisplaced No. 4
  and 5 phalanges
Advantage: Simple, inexpensive, can be
  applied by the patient, reasonable immobilization
Disadvantage: None
Cost: $1–2

Tube Splints

Use: Simple finger sprains
  Fractures: nondisplaced
  phalangeal
Advantage: Simple to put on;
  comfortable
Disadvantage: Expensive; may
  not sufficiently restrict motion
Cost: $15–16

Stax Splints

Use: Mallet finger
Fractures: tuft
Advantage: Inexpensive;
  easy to put on
Disadvantage: None
Cost: $3–4

HAND (cont.)

Dorsal Splint
Use: Mallet finger, minor finger
  sprains
Advantage: Easy to put on;
  inexpensive
Disadvantage: None
Cost: $2–3

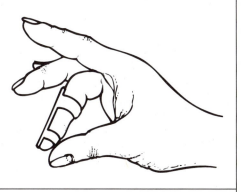

Metal Finger Splint
Use: Severe proximal interphalangeal or
  distal interphalangeal sprains
  Fractures: tuft fracture
Advantage: Better immobilization
  of the proximal interphalangeal
  joint; inexpensive
Disadvantage: Difficult to keep on;
  may irritate the palm
Cost : $3–4

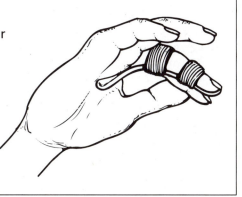

LUMBOSACRAL

Neoprene Waist Wrap
Use: Uncomplicated lumbosacral strain,
 facet syndrome, weightlifting
Advantage: Easy to put on; inexpensive;
 comfortable; can be easily worn
 under clothing; easily adjusted
Disadvantage: Insufficient support and
 immobilization
Cost: $12–15

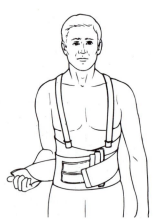

Velcro Lumbosacral Corset
Use: Lumbosacral strain, uncomplicated
 lumbosacral compression fracture,
 osteoarthritis, anklylosing spondylitis,
 recovery phase of lumbosacral
 radiculopathy, prevention of facet
 syndrome
Advantage: Easily put on; comfortable;
 relatively inexpensive; adjustable
Disadvantage: Insufficient support
 and immobilization
Cost: $15–20

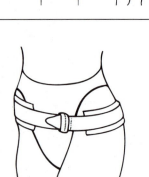

Elastic Sacroiliac Belt
Use: Sacroiliitis, iliolumbar syndrome,
 osteitis pubis, recovery phase of
 pelvic fracture
Advantage: Easy to put on; inexpensive;
 can be worn under clothing; easily adjusted
Disadvantage: Difficult to keep on if
 overweight; limited usefulness—variable
 patient response
Cost: $12–14

LUMBOSACRAL (cont.)

Lumbosacral Elastic Binder With Heated Plastic Shield
Use: Chronic low back pain, lumbosacral
  compression fracture, lumbosacral
  radiculopathy (healing phase)
Advantage: More support; maintains
  the lumbosacral spine in extension;
  more limitation of flexion
Disadvantage: Expensive; requires a
  technician to form the shield;
  not as comfortable
Cost: $125–135

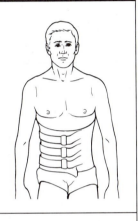

Three-Point Extension Brace (Jewett)
Use: Compression fractures,
  kyphosis from any cause
Advantage: Offers the greatest
  restriction of all braces
Disadvantage: Expensive; bulky and
  obtrusive; uncomfortable; not well
  tolerated; must be readjusted
  by a professional
Cost: $260–280

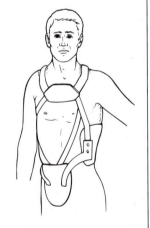

KNEE

Ace Wrap
Use: Any minor knee problem
Cost: $3–5

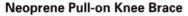

Neoprene Pull-on Knee Brace
Use: Osteoarthritis, prepatellar bursitis,
  first degree medial collateral ligament or
  lateral collateral ligament strain, Osgood-Schlatter
  disease, rheumatoid arthritis, bland knee effusions
Advantage: Easy to put on; inexpensive; simple
Disadvantage: Very little support; slips; hard
  to fit on obese patients; may restrict venous flow
Cost: Simple—$7–8;
  patellar cut out—$16–17

Velcro Knee Pads
Use: Prepatellar bursitis, infrapatellar
  bursitis, chondromalacia, patellofemoral
  osteoarthritis
Advantage: Plastic metal cup anterior is
  very protective; inexpensive; easy to put on
Disadvantage: May restrict venous blood flow
Cost: $15–20

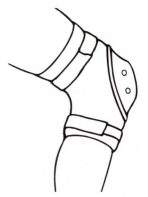

Patellar Strap
Use: Chondromalacia patella, patellar tendinitis,
  patellofemoral osteoarthritis, patellar subluxation,
  patellar dislocation
 Advantage: Simple; inexpensive;
  easy to put on and adjust
Disadvantage: May not provide enough correction
  of the abnormal patellofemoral tracking;
  may restrict venous blood flow
Cost: $15–16

KNEE (cont.)

Velcro Patellar Restraining Immobilizer
Use: Chondromalacia, patellar subluxation, patellar
  dislocation, patellofemoral osteoarthritis, first degree
  medial or lateral collateral ligament strains, osteoarthritis
Advantage: Improved patellofemoral tracking;
  easy to put on; patient acceptability
Disadvantage: Moderately expensive; hard to fit on
  obese patients
Cost: $35–37

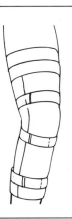

Velcro Straight Leg Brace
Use: Acute knee injury, second or third degree medial
  or lateral collateral ligament strains, patellar tendinitis,
  medical management of a meniscus tear
Advantage: Excellent protection and immobilization
  of the knee; easily put on
Disadvantage: Relatively expensive; bulky; cannot wear
  under clothing; affects normal walking gait
Cost: 18"— $36–38
  24"— $44–46

Metal Hinged Braces (McDavid Knee Guard), Lenox Hill Derotational Brace, Don Joy Rehabilitation Brace
Use: Ligament instability (especially anterior cruciate
  ligament), postoperative anterior cruciate ligament
  repair, third degree medial or lateral collateral ligament
  instability, osteoarthritis with angulation, hyperextension
  laxity
Advantage: Excellent and variable control of knee motion
  and immobilization; better varus/vagus protection
Disadvantage: Very expensive; custom-made; not
  readily available
Cost: $800-900

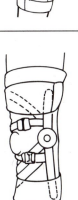

ANKLE

Neoprene Pull-on Ankle Brace
Use: Minor sprains, minor degrees of pronation,
  mild osteoarthritis
Advantage: Simple; inexpensive;
  relatively easy to put on
Disadvantage: Hard to wear in a shoe;
  not very supportive
Cost: $7–8

New Skin/Moleskin
Use: Achilles tendinitis, pre-Achilles bursitis,
  bursitis over bunions, dorsal bunion,
  blisters/abrasions
Advantage: Easy to apply; inexpensive;
  can be custom-cut to shape or size
Disadvantage: None
Cost: $2–3

Velcro Ankle Brace
Use: Recurrent ankle sprain, osteoarthritis of the ankle,
  moderate pronation, posterior tibialis tenosynovitis,
  peroneus tenosynovitis, tarsal tunnel
Advantage: Easy to put on; relatively inexpensive;
  better support than a neoprene pull-on
Disadvantage: Still does not provide adequate
  support for some conditions
Cost: $29–32

ANKLE (cont.)

Rocker-bottom Plastic Ankle immobilizer
Use: Achilles tendinitis, severe ankle sprain, posterior
 tibialis tenosynovitis, peroneus tenosynovitis, severe
 plantar fasciitis, stress fracture of the foot
Advantage: Excellent support and restriction of the ankle;
 removable; comfortable
Disadvantage: Expensive; bulky; difficult to drive a car
Cost: $54–58

Short Leg Walking Cast
Use: Achilles tendinitis, severe ankle sprain,
 plantar fasciitis, severe flare of ankle arthritis,
 stress fracture of the heel or metatarsal
 Fractures: nondisplaced bimalleolar,
 nondisplaced fibular
Advantage: Excellent immobilization;
 the patient cannot remove it
Disadvantage: Expensive; cannot drive
 safely; bulky; may throw off walking gait;
 cannot get it wet; requires a technician
Cost: Plaster—$51–54; fiberglass—$94–100

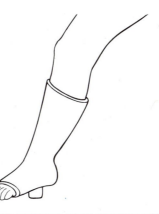

Unna Boot
Use: Venous stasis ulcer, moderate
 ankle sprain, poorly healing wounds
 Fractures: minimally displaced fibular
Advantage: Lightweight; requires a technician
Disadvantage: Does not sufficiently immobilize
 or protect the ankle; cannot get it wet
Cost: $21–22 versus
 athletic tape—$4–5

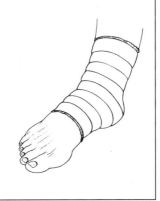

ANKLE (cont.)

Footdrop Night Splint, Ready-Made
Ankle Foot Orthosis, Custom-Made
Ankle Foot Orthosis
Use: Stroke, Charcot-Marie-Tooth
   disease, polio or post polio, any
   cause of footdrop
Advantage: Protects against
   flexion contractures; improves gait;
   prevents falls
Disadvantage: None
Cost: $15–40
   (depending if it is custom-made or not)

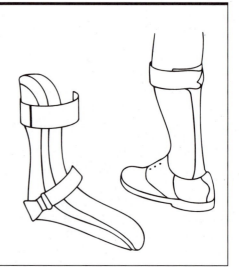

FOOT

Heel Cushions
Use: Heel pad syndrome, plantar
  fasciitis/spur, calcaneal stress fracture,
  ankle arthritis
Advantage: Inexpensive; effective
  cushioning of the heel; transferable
  from one shoe to another; doesn't wear out
Disadvantage: Won't correct an arch
  problem or an alignment problem of
  the ankle
Cost: $3–5

Heel Cups
Use: Heel pad syndrome, plantar fasciitis/spur,
  calcaneal stress fracture, severe
  epiphysiitis, hip or knee osteoarthritis
Advantage: Inexpensive; effective
  cushioning of the heel; transferable
  from one shoe to another
Disadvantage: Won't correct an arch
  problem or an alignment problem
  of the ankle
Cost: $5–8

Padded Insoles (Spenco or Sorbothane)
Use: Heel pad syndrome, hammer toes, calluses, metatarsalgia, rheumatoid
  disease of the metatarsophalangeals, Morton neuroma, ankle, knee, or hip
  osteoarthritis, healing phase of stress fractures of the foot
Advantage: Excellent cushioning of the entire foot;
  inexpensive; transferable from one
  shoe to another
Disadvantage: Does not have
  an arch support
Cost: $8–12

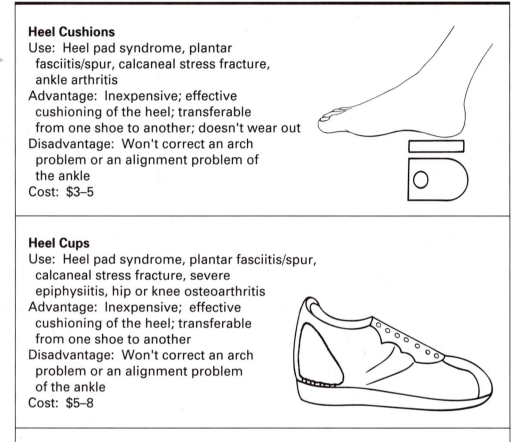

FOOT (cont.)

Padded Insoles With Arch Supports
Use: Plantar fasciitis, pes cavus, pes planus,
  pronated ankles, tarsal tunnel
Advantage: Soft padding plus arch support;
  relatively inexpensive; transferable
  from one shoe to another
Disadvantage: Not enough
  arch support to
  correct moderate to
  severe arch abnormalities
Cost: $18–22

**Plastic Orthotic Arch Supports
(Over The Counter or Custom-Made)**
Use: Persistent plantar fasciitis, pes cavus,
  pes planus, ankle pronation, tarsal tunnel
Advantage: Can correct any degree
  of arch abnormality
Disadvantage: Expensive; must
  be custom-made; time delay to
  obtain; hard surface without any padding
Cost: Over the counter—$25–28; custom fit —$75–95

Bunion Shields
Use: Bunions
Advantage: Provides protection to the soft
  tissues and the joint; inexpensive
Disadvantage: None
Cost: $4–5

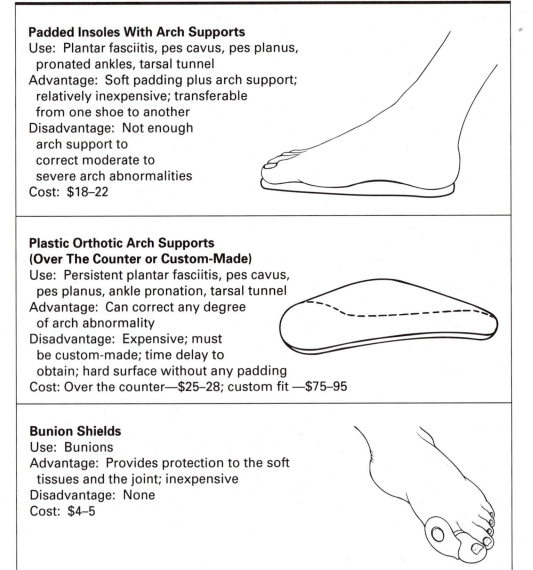

FOOT (cont.)

Metatarsal Bar
Use: Stress fracture of the metatarsal,
 Fractures: nondisplaced phalangeal,
 nondisplaced metatarsal
Advantage: Reduced pressure over
 the forefoot
Disadvantage: Shoes have to be
 altered; may throw off normal
 walking gait; can be expensive
 if many shoes are adjusted
Cost: $20–25

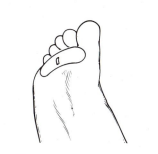

Hammer Toe Crests
Use: Hammer toes
Advantage: Easy to put on; inexpensive
Disadvantage: Mildly uncomfortable
Cost: $12–14

Felt Rings
 Use: Bunion of the first metatarsophalangeal,
 dorsal bunion, corns, calluses, hammer toes,
 pre-Achilles bursitis
Advantage: Easy to apply; inexpensive
Disadvantage: Skin rash from the
 adhesive (rare)
Cost: $2–3

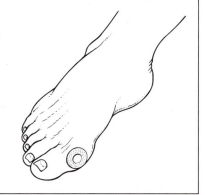

FOOT (cont.)

Toe Spacers, Cotton or Plastic
Use: Morton neuroma, interdigital
  soft corns, bunions, any toe deformity
Advantage: Easy to apply; inexpensive
Disadvantage: None
Cost: Cotton—$1–2;
  rubber—$2–3

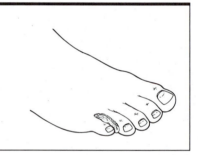

Appendix

Nonsteroidal Anti-Inflammatory Drugs

Generic	Trade	Dose (max daily)	Cost per 100 in Dollars
Salicylates			
Acetylsalicylic acid*	Anacin, Ascriptin, Bufferin, Ecotrin	325,500(5–6 g)	4–5
Choline magnesium trisalicylate	Trilisate	0.5,0.75,1 g(3 g)	77–80
Diflunisal	Dolobid	250,500(1500)	95–117
Salsalate*	Disalcid, Salsitab	500,750(3000)	16–22
Proprionic acids			
Fenoprofen calcium	Nalfon	200,300,600(3200)	57–87
Flurbiprofen	Ansaid	50,100(300)	83–124
Ibuprofen*	Advil, Motrin, Nuprin, Rufen	200,400,600,800(3000)	5–18
Ketoprofen	Orudis	25,50,75(300)	90–120
Naproxen	Naprosyn	250,375,500(1500)	62–122
Naproxen sodium	Anaprox	275,550(1650)	81–121
Acetic acids			
Diclofenac sodium	Voltaren	25,50,75(200)	54–116
Indomethacin*	Indocin	25,50,75SR(200)	20–32
Nabumetone	Relafen	500,750(2000)	99–130
Sulindac*	Clinoril	150,200(400)	82–96
Tolmetin sodium	Tolectin	200,400(1800)	22–61
Oxicams			
Piroxicam	Feldene	10,20(20)	100–214
Fenamates			
Meclofenamate sodium*	Meclomen	50,100(400)	24–44
Mefenamic acid	Ponstel	250(500)	91–94
Pyranocarboxylic acid			
Etodolac	Lodine	200,300(1200)	99–110
Pyrrolopyrrole			
Ketorolac	Toradol	15,30,60(120–150)	117–120
Pyrazolones			
Phenylbutazone	Butazolidin	100(400)	27–30

*Available in generic form

Corticosteroids

Corticosteroid	Trade Name Abbreviation	Strength (mg/ml)	Equivalent Milligrams of Hydrocortisone
SHORT-ACTING PREPARATIONS (soluble)			
Hydrocortisone phosphate (Hydrocortone phosphate)	H	25, 50	25, 50
Prednisolone (Hydeltrasol injection)	H20	20	80
LONG-ACTING PREPARATIONS (depot/time released)			
Triamcinolone acetonide (Kenalog)	K40	40	200
Triamcinolone hexacetonide (Aristospan)	A20	20	100
Methylprednisolone acetate (Depo-Medrol)	D80	20, 40, 80	100–300
Dexamethasone phosphate (Decadron)	Dex8	4, 8	100, 200
Prednisolone tebutate (Hydeltra-TBA)	HTBA	20	80
COMBINATION PREPARATIONS (both soluble and depot)			
Betamethasone sodium phosphate (Celestone Soluspan)	C6	6	150

Calcium Supplementation

	Amount or Tablet Size	Calcium Content (mg)	Annual Cost (dollars)
FOODS			
Milk (nonfat)	1 cup	290–300	200
Yogurt	1 cup	240–400	950
Cheese slice	1 oz	160–260	260
Cottage cheese	½ cup	80–100	960
Broccoli	1 cup	160–180	2000
Tofu	4 oz	145–155	1500
Salmon, canned	3 oz	170–200	3700
SUPPLEMENTS			
Calcium carbonate			
Oyster shell (generic)	625, 1250, 1500	250, 500, 600	40
Os-Cal	625, 1250	250, 500	108
Os-Cal + D	625, 1250	250, 500	107
Tum-Ex	750	300	55
Calcium-rich Rolaids	550	220	53
Caltrate	1500	600	108
Caltrate + D (125u)	1500	600	108
Calcium phosphate			
Posture	1565	600	115
Posture D (125u)	1565	600	115
Calcium lactate	650	85	350
Calcium gluconate	975	90	522
Calcium citrate			
Citracal 950	950	200	162
Citracal 1500 + (200u)	1500	315	162

REFERENCES

History

Hollander JL, Brown EM, Jessar RA, and Brown CY: Hydrocortisone and cortisone injected into arthritic joints: Comparative effects of and use of hydrocortisone as a local antiarthritic. JAMA 147:1929–1635, 1951.

Hollander and associates in Philadelphia are the first to describe the usefulness of locally administered hydrocortisone injected into arthritic joints.

Lapidus PW and Guidotti FP: Local injections of hydrocortisone in 495 orthopedic patients. Industr Med Surg 26:234–244, 1957.

Lapidus, who is an orthopedic surgeon practicing in New York city, describes the beneficial effects of injectable hydrocortisone when used to treat outpatient orthopedic conditions (e.g., shoulder tendinitis, olecranon bursitis, trigger finger).

Numerous articles in the late 1960s and early 1970s.

The long-acting depot esters of hydrocortisone are developed and introduced (e.g, triamcinolone, methylprednisolone, betamethasone, and dexamethasone). Many studies demonstrate the usefulness of these drugs in treating articular and orthopedic problems.

Use

Ellis RM, Hollingworth GR, and MacCollum MS: Comparison of injection techniques for shoulder pain: Results of a double-blind, randomized study. BMJ 287:1339–1341, 1983.

In this double-blind, randomized study, Ellis and co-workers demonstrate the importance of local injection technique. The local trigger point injection was inferior to an "anatomically placed" corticosteroid injection when treating shoulder tendinitis and capsulitis.

White RH, Paull DM, and Fleming KW: Rotator cuff tendinitis: Comparison of subacromial injection of a long-acting corticosteroid versus oral indomethacin therapy. J Rheum 13:608–613, 1986.

This double-blind, prospective study of 40 patients showed the efficacy of oral nonsteroidal therapy to be equal to the efficacy of local corticosteroid injection when treating shoulder tendinitis.

Day BH and Gavindasamy N: Corticosteroid injection in the treatment of tennis elbow. Pract Med 220:459–462, 1978.

Local injection of methylprednisolone for tennis elbow is highly effective when compared with Xylocaine or Saline alone ($P<.001$). Ninety per cent of patients responded to the local injection in this double-blind study.

Gray RG, Kiem IM, and Gottlieb NL: Intratendon sheath corticosteroid treatment of rheumatoid arthritis-associated and idiopathic flexor tenosynovitis. Arthritis Rheum 21:92–96, 1978.

The long-acting depot corticosteroid drugs differ in efficacy. In treating trigger finger in rheumatoid arthritis and non-rheumatoid arthritis patients, significant differences in response were noted among triamcinolone, betamethasone, and prednisolone tertiary-butyl-acetate. Triamcinolone provided the best overall response.

Anderson BC, Manthey R, and Brouns MC: Treatment of de Quervain's tenosynovitis with corticosteroids. Arthritis Rheum 34:793–798, 1991.

The preferred treatment of de Quervain tenosynovitis is a local injection of a long-acting corticosteroid derivative. Ninety per cent of 56 cases (the largest prospective study in the literature) were effectively managed with local injection. Adverse reactions were minor, and relief was long-lasting (see the accompanying editorial).

Anderson BC and Kaye S: Treatment of flexor tenosynovitis of the hand ("trigger finger") with corticosteroids. Arch Intern Med 151:153–156, 1991.

Local injection of trigger finger is effective in nearly 90% of cases, provides long-lasting relief over years, and is free from serious adverse reactions.

Phalen GS: Carpel tunnel syndrome: 17 years of experience in diagnosis and treatment. J Bone Joint Surg 48A:211–228, 1966.

Ninety per cent of patients with carpal tunnel syndrome respond to splinting and to local corticosteroid injection

Foster JB and Goodman HV: The effect of local corticosteroid injection on median nerve conduction in carpal tunnel syndrome. Ann Phys Med 6:287–294, 1962.

Eight-five per cent of patients with carpal tunnel syndrome respond to injection at 6 weeks. At 12 to 18 months, only 30% of patients maintain that improvement.

Boyd HB and McLeod AC: Tennis elbow. J Bone Joint Surg 55A:1183–1197, 1973.

Of 871 cases with tennis elbow, only 5% fail conservative treatment and require surgery.

Seminars in Arthritis and Rheumatism. May, 1981.

This is a comprehensive review of the indications, use, adverse reactions, and pharmacology of the injectable corticosteroids. The long-acting esters (especially triamcinolone) provide significantly longer benefit than does hydrocortisone.

Complications

Hollander JL, Jessar RA, and Brown EM: Intra-synovial corticosteroid therapy: A decade of use. Bull Rheum Dis 11:239–240, 1961.

Over a 10-year period, Hollander and associates performed over 100,000 intra-articular injections. Fourteen cases of local postinjection infection occurred for a rate of 1 per 7000 procedures.

Kendall PH: Untoward effects following local hydrocortisone injection. Ann Phys Med 4:170–175, 1961.

Kendall performed 6700 hydrocortisone injections over a 3-year period in 2256 patients. Only 73 significant reactions occurred, including four cases of infection (6 per 10,000), allergic reactions, minor bleeding, nausea and vomiting, and local weakness. He did not describe any postinjection tissue disruption.

Ismail AM, Balakrishnan R, and Rajakumar MK: Rupture of patellar ligament after steroid infiltration: Report of a case. J Bone Joint Surg 51B:503–505, 1969.
Bedi SS and Ellis W: Spontaneous rupture of the calcaneal tendon in rheumatoid arthritis after steroid injection. Ann Rheum Dis 29:494–495, 1970.
Kleinman M and Gross AE: Achilles tendon rupture following steroid injection. J Bone Joint Surg 65A:1345–1347, 1983.

Postinjection tendon rupture has been described. Most of the literature from the 1960s and 1970s describes case reports that consist almost exclusively of patients with connective tissue disorders. The exact relationship between tendon rupture and corticosteroid injection remains controversial. Tendon rupture in the small tendons following local injection has not been described. Only patellar, Achilles, biceps, and rotator cuff tendon ruptures have been described following injection. These tendons are known to spontaneously rupture as well!

Personal Unpublished Data

The most predictable side effects from local injection are subcutaneous atrophy and postinjection inflammatory flare. Atrophy is seen almost exclusively in the upper extremity (e.g., tennis elbow, de Quervain, dorsal ganglion). Triamcinolone is four times as likely as Depo-Medrol to cause subcutaneous atrophy. This cosmetic effect almost always resolves after 6 to 9 months.

Depo-Medrol is twice as likely as triamcinolone to cause postinjection swelling and pain. When performing an injection, the patient must be warned against atrophy and 2 to 3 days of increased discomfort.

Index